Doctors and Patients

An Anthology

Edited by
Cecil Helman

Radcliffe Medical Press

Radcliffe Medical Press Ltd
18 Marcham Road
Abingdon
Oxon OX14 1AA
United Kingdom

www.radcliffe-oxford.com
The Radcliffe Medical Press electronic catalogue and online ordering facility.
Direct sales to anywhere in the world.

British Library Cataloguing in Publication Data

A catalogue record for this book is available from the British Library.

ISBN 1 85775 993 1

Typeset by Advance Typesetting Ltd, Oxfordshire
Printed and bound by TJ International Ltd, Padstow, Cornwall

Contents

About the editor

Cecil Helman was born in 1944 in Cape Town, South Africa, and now lives in London. He is both a doctor and a writer, and also has a degree in anthropology. His books, translated into six languages, include: a collection of short stories, *The Exploding Newspaper & Other Fables*; a book of essays, *Body Myths* (published in the USA as *The Body of Frankenstein's Monster: essays in myth and medicine*); and a textbook, *Culture, Health and Illness*. His short stories and prose poems have been included in ten anthologies – and in many literary magazines – in the USA, Britain and South Africa. In 1983–84, he was a Visiting Fellow in Social Medicine and Health Policy, at Harvard Medical School. Currently he is Associate Professor of Medical Anthropology at Brunel University, and Senior Lecturer in the Department of Primary Care and Population Sciences, Royal Free and University College Medical School.

Acknowledgements

The editor would like to acknowledge the following publishers, agents and authors for rights to reprint these stories:

- *Baptism by Rotation* by Mikhail Bulgakov, from *A Country Doctor's Notebook*, translated by Michael Glenny, published by Collins-Harvill. Reprinted by permission of The Random House Group Ltd.

- *Baptism by Rotation* by Mikhail Bulgakov, from *A Country Doctor's Notebook*, translated by Michael Glenny, published by Collins-Harvill. © Mikhail Bulgakov – translated by Michael Glenny. Reproduced by permission of Rogers, Coleridge & White Ltd, 20 Powis Mews, London W11 1JN.

- *A Doctor's Visit* by Anton Chekhov, from *The Lady With the Dog and Other Stories*, translated by Constance Garnett. Used by permission of AP Watt Ltd, on behalf of the Executor of the Estate of Constance Garnett.

- *Inside Out and Upside Down: diagnosis* by Rachel Clark, from Clark R with Jefferies N, Hasler J and Pendleton D (2002) *A Long Walk Home*. Radcliffe Medical Press, Oxford. © 2002 Rachel Clark/Naomi Jefferies. Reprinted by permission of Naomi Jefferies.

- *The Case of David Murray* by AJ Cronin, from *Adventures in Two Worlds*. Reprinted by permission of Victor Gollancz Ltd, a division of The Orion Publishing Group Ltd.

- *The Case of David Murray* by AJ Cronin, from *Adventures in Two Worlds*. © AJ Cronin. Reprinted by permission of AM Heath & Co Ltd.

- *A Medical Document* by Arthur Conan Doyle, from *Tales of Adventure and Medical Life* (John Murray, 1963). First published in 1922.

- *The Other Half of Eddie Barnett* by Cecil Helman, from the *London Magazine* **36**(7,8), October–November, 1996.

- *Let Me Feel Your Pulse* by O Henry, from *The Best of O Henry* (Hodder & Stoughton, 1954).

- *A Country Doctor* by Franz Kafka, translated by Iain Bamforth. Published in 1999 by the *British Journal of General Practice*. **49**: 1036–9. Used by permission of the *British Journal of General Practice*.

- *Sanatorium* by W Somerset Maugham. From *The Complete Short Stories by W Somerset Maugham* published by William Heinemann, 1951. Reprinted by permission of The Random House Group Ltd.

- *Observer Life*, 3 August 1997, column by Ruth Picardie, from *Before I Say Goodbye* by Ruth Picardie with Matt Seaton and Justine Picardie (Penguin Books, 1998). © 1997 Ruth Picardie. *Observer Life* columns © 1997 Ruth Picardie and Justine Picardie.

- *In the Gray Zone*, from *My Grandfather's Blessings* by Rachel Naomi Remen MD. © 2000 by Rachel Naomi Remen MD. Used by permission of Riverhead Books, a division of Penguin Putnam, Inc.

- *Telling the Truth* by Renate Rubinstein, from *Take It and Leave It: aspects of being ill* by Renate Rubinstein, translated by Karin Fierke and Aad Janssen (Marion Boyars Publishers, 1985). Reprinted by permission of Marion Boyars Publishers Ltd, London.

- *Rebecca* by Oliver Sacks, from *The Man Who Mistook His Wife For a Hat* (Picador, 1985). © 1985 by Oliver Sacks. Reprinted by permission of The Wylie Agency, Inc.

- *The King of Xingu* by Moacyr Scliar. Adapted and translated from Portuguese by the author. Reprinted by permission of the author. Extract taken from *A Majestado do Xingu*, first published by Companhia das Letras, Sao Paolo, Brazil, in 1997.

- *My Life as a Pig* by Clive Sinclair, from *A Soap Opera From Hell* (Picador). © 1998 Clive Sinclair. Reproduced by permission of Rogers, Coleridge & White Ltd, 20 Powis Mews, London W11 1JN.

- *The Use of Force* by William Carlos Williams, from *The Collected Stories of William Carlos Williams*. © 1938 by William Carlos Williams. Reprinted by permission of New Directions Publishing Corp.

- *The Use of Force* by William Carlos Williams, from *Collected Poems* (2000) by William Carlos Williams. Reprinted by permission of Carcanet Press Ltd.

Notes

- If there are any errors or omissions in this list, they will be corrected in future reprints of this book.

- *A Doctor's Visit* by Anton Chekhov is from *The Lady With the Dog and Other Stories* (Chatto and Windus, 1917), in the translation by Constance Garnett.

- The quotes from the poems by Raphael Campo and Danny Abse are taken from *Blood & Bone: poems by physicians*, edited by Angela Belli and Jack Coulehan (University of Iowa Press, 1998).

- I am particularly grateful to three friends of mine – Oliver Sacks, Clive Sinclair and Moacyr Scliar – for permission to include their stories in this book.

Dedication

To my daughter Zoe.

Introduction: The Healing Bond

by Cecil Helman

This anthology celebrates one of the most unique, but also problematic, forms of human relationship: that between an ill person and their doctor. All the stories within it – both autobiography and fiction – have been chosen to illustrate different aspects of this singular but universal relationship.

The stories that follow describe two distinct but inter-related worlds, and how – in hospitals and homes, in clinics and surgeries and sanatoria – they interact with one another at times of human suffering. Some illustrate the more positive aspects of that relationship: empathy, kindness, attention and the curing of disease. But in others, the relationship is much more complex and ambivalent, even hostile, the encounter charged with anxiety and apprehension, as well as with hope.

In every human life, doctors wait in the wings. Encountering one of them is a situation that almost everyone will experience, usually reluctantly, at one time or another. Patients and their doctors are forever bound tightly together – whether they like it or not.

In compiling this collection, I have tried to select pieces that not only have literary merit, but which also shed light on how *differently* illness can be viewed from opposite sides of the sick bed, or of the doctor's desk. For this reason, the stories in the first part of the book – including those by Arthur Conan Doyle, Mikhail Bulgakov and Rachel Remen – are written mainly from the doctor's perspective, while those in the second part are mainly autobiographical texts – written by people who have experienced a serious, life-threatening disease: in this case, cancer, kidney failure and multiple sclerosis. A third group of stories looks more closely at some clinical encounters between the two parties, and the interplay of personalities at this crucial moment.

This anthology, then, is a celebration – sometimes a nostalgic one – of a unique and archetypal relationship: a *healing bond* between doctor and patient. One that has always existed, and always will.

In our modern technological world, however, this relationship is changing rapidly. And as many of these stories show, for patients – as well as for doctors – not all those changes have been positive.

Medical stories

'There's no need for fiction in medicine,' remarks Foster, the general practitioner in Arthur Conan Doyle's story, 'for the facts will always beat anything you can fancy.' In fact, medicine *is* all about stories. About the stories of patient and doctor, and how in their clinical encounters these stories mingle or diverge. The patient's 'history', the doctor's 'diagnosis' or 'prognosis', are all part of the same process – a shared way of understanding human misfortune, and then trying to deal with it. A way of giving it a shape and a form: a name, an identity.

Perhaps that is why most doctors are natural story tellers. Wherever a group of doctors gather together informally, as in Conan Doyle's *A Medical Document*, their tales of patients – often thinly disguised as 'interesting cases' – are part of the folk culture of the medical profession: their black humour often puzzling, and sometimes repellent, to the outsider. But for many doctors, story telling itself is an essential part of their lives. Often it can play an important psychological role: as a form of informal therapy – or rather, of group therapy. Such ironic stories can be a way of *making sense* of their daily experience of human suffering, a way of giving it meaning. Of keeping despair and death at bay.

A few of these medical stories form a special sub-genre of their own. These are the narratives of their most difficult patients, the ones with impossible symptoms or unbelievable complaints. Like the denizens of some medieval bestiary, these bizarre or hypochondriacal patients – often called 'heartsink' or 'fat file' patients – are compared, wondered at and minutely discussed, often with the tiniest shudder. Conan Doyle's story captures this atmosphere of medical story telling, and shows how the doctors' stories interlock and overlap, following one another in a sort of rhythm, almost like a barber shop song. Story after story, round and around. 'That's the worst of these medical stories –' complains the outsider, listening in, 'they never seem to have an end.'

It is no coincidence, therefore, that so many doctors have themselves become writers (one website, for example, lists no fewer than 300 of them, ranging from Rabelais to Celine, Kobo Abe to Oliver Goldsmith, Tobias Smollett to Michael Crichton). Or that over half the pieces in this collection are actually by physician-writers: Sacks, Scliar, Maugham, Conan Doyle, Cronin, Helman, Williams, Bulgakov and Chekhov. In each case, the fact that the authors are – or were – medical doctors themselves gives their narratives a special, knowing atmosphere, and a particular quality of authenticity.

Patients versus people

The second part of this anthology comprises a collection of patients' narratives – what Howard Brody calls 'stories of suffering' – as well as two fictional pieces. Never mawkish or self-pitying, the autobiographical pieces deal mostly with severe, progressive diseases. They show that for seriously ill people – as with doctors – telling the story of one's illness can be a way of unifying experience, of imposing some sense of coherence on to the chaos that is sudden, unexpected, life-threatening disease. It enables one not only to share that experience with others, but also to distil some personal meaning from it.

All these personal narratives cluster around a central focus: *the disease*. How it began, how it arrived and declared itself, how it was treated, and how it then progressed or retreated. And particularly how it so completely transformed the patient's life. They show how such illnesses can radically and irreversibly change one's perceptions – especially of oneself.

They also illustrate that every episode of illness is unique. And that within the role of 'patient', no one ever experiences the same illness in *exactly* the same way. For the identical symptoms can mean very different things to different people. And each ill person always gives subtly different answers to those two key questions, when illness strikes: 'Why has it happened to *me*?' and 'Why *now*?'

But they also show some fundamental differences: between the perspectives of patients and those of their doctors; and between the patient's individual experience of suffering, and the more formal, generalised models of disease used by their doctors. It is a problem that is present in all forms of healing.

Although in his book *The Healer's Art*, the New York physician Eric J Cassell has remarked that, ideally, 'doctors do not treat disease; they treat patients who have diseases', some of these narratives suggest a rather different picture. They give an image of high-tech hospital settings where something crucial, some human singularity, has been lost from the doctor–patient relationship. Finding themselves faced with a dangerous illness, several of the narrators find themselves being regarded merely as a disease, or as a diseased organ – their body fragmented and depersonalised, divided up among many different medical specialities.

Renate Rubinstein, for example, protests against the way some doctors define a person mainly by their disease ('disabled' or 'a cancer victim'). She rejects, too, those who blame her own multiple sclerosis on her 'pathological personality'. In the past (as Susan Sontag points out in her *Illness as Metaphor*), many other chronic, incurable conditions have been explained in this way, including cancer and tuberculosis (TB). Such diseases, difficult to treat or identify, have often been blamed on the patient – or, more recently, on their 'unexpressed emotions', such as anger or grief, echoing the remark of the 19th-century anatomist Henry Maudsley that 'the sorrow that has no vent in tears, makes other organs weep'. In this view, the disease you get is typical of who you really are – and you, in turn, are typical of the disease. In the 19th century, TB was often seen as a symptom of refinement and over-sensitivity, but as Rubinstein ironically points out, despite the fact that Chekhov suffered from TB for the last decade of his life, no one today would ever dream of saying – after seeing one of his plays – that they were written by a 'typical tuberculosis patient'.

But severe life-threatening illnesses *can* redefine one, in a very unwelcome way. For one thing, they can suddenly propel you into the centre of attention and make you the object of interest, compassion, pity or wonder. Illness can force you to reflect on your life, past and future, in a way that you never did before. In Somerset Maugham's *Sanatorium*, one Henry Chester, an ordinary man, 'born and bred to lead an average life, exposed to the normal vicissitudes of existence', finds himself if not ennobled by his fatal tuberculosis, then at least growing in self-awareness as a result of it.

From the doctor's perspective, then, the challenge is to keep sight of the person, hidden beneath the diagnosis. In Oliver Sacks's *Rebecca*, the neurologist notices for the first time the young handicapped girl, so severely disabled, sunning herself happily outside his clinic on a warm spring day. For the first time he glimpses – with 'my human, as opposed to my neurological vision' – the person within the handicap. The one that lives happily there, in poetry and in narrative. Until that moment, he writes, all his neurological and psychological tests were designed 'not merely to uncover, to bring out her deficits, but to decompose her into functions and deficits'.

Medicine and machines

Dr Korolyov, in Chekhov's *A Doctor's Visit*, relies for his understanding of the young girl's problem not on any fancy diagnostic equipment, but rather on his own powers of observation, his intuition and empathy. His story reminds one that, until quite recently, a doctor's diagnosis relied primarily on the *human* senses – not on technology. Even in the 1960s, when I was a medical student in South Africa, the emphasis was still on examining patients and making a diagnosis by using *all* your senses: sight, touch, hearing and smell, as well as memory. The use of diagnostic technology – such as x-rays or blood tests – was important then, but was never expected to tell the whole story. What was more important was what you saw, what you heard, what you felt with your fingertips, and even the smell of the patient's body or breath. The sickly-sweet breath of the severe diabetic, say, or the dullness in a congested chest when you tapped it with your fingertips. When examining a patient's chest, the mantra of our teachers was: *inspection – palpation – percussion – auscultation*. You looked at the chest, felt it as it breathed, tapped it – and only then did you listen to it through your stethoscope. It was a diagnostic process made mainly between two people: doctor and patient.

But these days, a third presence – shiny, metallic and ubiquitous – has made its appearance in the doctor–patient relationship: whirring and pulsating at the patient's bedside or in the doctor's office. The monitor machine, the x-ray, the MRI (magnetic resonance imaging) or CAT (computed axial tomography) scan have all become more than mere tools of the doctor's trade. In some ways, they have also become a new type of inanimate healer themselves. In most patients' stories of suffering, they now play a greater role than they ever did before.

Medical technology enables one to see secrets hidden below the skin. The devices can peer deep inside you, revealing disease at the tiniest, most invisible level: cells, enzymes, bodily fluids, even molecules. For the first time in human history, the body has become transparent to the human gaze. But at the same time, technology can make it more mysterious. Where, after all, is the *person* on the x-ray plate – that pre-cognitive photograph of the future? Knowing everything about someone's skeleton tells us nothing about who its owner is: their needs and fears and hopes, their prejudices and beliefs.

In 1983, even the prestigious *Journal of the American Medical Association* sounded a warning bell, deploring the growing development of a medical system that had become so impersonal and dominated by technology, and felt obliged to ask the question, 'Has the machine become the physician?':

> The fact that the health care provided in the system may be improved as a result of the technology does not have as much impact as the subtle and hidden message that the machine has become the physician: the definitive adviser. The specialist-physician is metamorphosing into a technocrat and a businessman. The physician retreats behind the machine, and becomes an extension of the machine.

Increasingly, some patients *also* find themselves becoming an extension of a machine. In Clive Sinclair's story *My Life as a Pig*, the renal dialysis machine becomes a part of him, an extension of his body. Like a new, extra organ, it extends his body far beyond its natural borders of skin. Medical machines like that can blur the boundaries of who we are, and can change fundamentally our sense of self.

Nature and time

Unlike the machine-based medicine of today, many of the earlier stories in this book – such as those by Conan Doyle, Maugham and Chekhov – tell of an age where *nature* was seen as one of the causes of diseases (especially of respiratory diseases). Draughts, chills, damp, heat, the dirty air or *miasms* of the overcrowded cities were all seen as contributing to disease, despite the development of germ theory. But nature was also seen as part of the *cure* – especially in alliance with the human body and the human spirit. In certain environments – such as the cool and pellucid air of the Alps, or the dry desert air of Arizona – nature itself would effect most of the cure. 'Fresh air', sea, wind, water and sun were all believed to have healing properties.

In many of these stories, the reader will also note how *time* plays a similar role. For it is Time, as a force of Nature, that is the true healer, and the wise doctor works in alliance with it. 'The art of medicine,' once wrote the sardonic Voltaire, 'consists in amusing the patient while nature cures the disease.'

The patients in Somerset Maugham's *Sanatorium* (like those in Thomas Mann's novel *The Magic Mountain*) float in a timeless zone. They are citizens of a tiny planet, orbiting free of many of the usual constraints of everyday life. They form a small community of suffering, a distorted reflection of the world outside. Ashenden, the new arrival, finds it to be a miniature society, with its own feuds and rivalries, its deep friendships and burgeoning love affairs. Within the sanatorium, each patient occupies themselves with their own private battle against tuberculosis. The only treatments on offer are not miracle drugs, but rather rest, fresh air, exercise, good food and sunshine – and, of course, *time*. Time that stretches on and on, healing some, destroying others.

In other settings (as in my own story, *The Other Half of Eddie Barnett*), time can also reveal the true diagnosis, as well as suggest the best form of treatment. But in many of the patient narratives, time flows swiftly in another direction. Time, like the Goddess Kali, is the destroyer of life. Each day, in the narratives by Ruth Picardie and Rachel Clark, the disease advances inexorably, conquering more and more territory within their bodies. For Renate Rubinstein, with her multiple sclerosis, time seems to advance fitfully, sometimes retreating for a while, but nevertheless taking away one bit of her bodily functioning (and independence) after another. In Clive Sinclair's story, the kidney transplant he undergoes reverses the downward spiral of time. From the transplant operation a new composite body is formed, a living hybrid of two histories, a sort of secular life after death.

This slow march of time, either forwards or backwards, is the very opposite of the rapid, urgent sense of time portrayed in popular medical TV dramas, such as *ER*. In the hubbub of the emergency room, time is seen as compressed, condensed into the intense moment, as the green-gowned heroes and heroines battle weekly with the forces of disease and death. In *ER*, sick strangers come and go, entering through one door, then exiting through another. Before they leave – either admitted to the hospital or wheeled away to the morgue – there are brief, poignant glimpses of their human frailty. As in much of modern hospital medicine, there is no time for the patients to form a community of their own, as they do in *Sanatorium*: only the doctors have time for that. One of the attractions of TV programmes like this is to show that some sense of order *can*, after all, be imposed on the chaos of inner-city life – at least for the briefest moment.

Practising in a speeded-up world, relying more on machines than on the rhythms of nature, many modern doctors now find themselves searching for a 'quick fix' for all medical problems. And many of their patients, too, have now become *im*patients – endlessly dissatisfied with their medical care, as they wait restlessly for that 'quick fix' to arrive.

Generalists versus specialists

In the stories by Williams, Conan Doyle, Bulgakov, Chekhov and Kafka – mostly written early last century – the hero is the *generalist*: the general practitioner, or the country doctor. A physician right in the front line of medical care. Someone who is exposed, day and night, to the raw material of human suffering. Who never knows who, or what, might walk through their office door next; or – as in Bulgakov's story – arrive at their clinic in the middle of a stormy night. Similarly, for the busy inner-city GP, a mass of suffering humanity pours through the door every day, chaotic and unsorted: patients of every age and type, and with every possible disorder. The generalist's role, in this situation, is not only to treat, but also to *sort*: mild cases from severe ones, really ill people from the 'worried well', the treatable from the doomed.

In Conan Doyle's *A Medical Document*, each of the three medical men swapping stories represents a common type (or rather stereotype) of 19th- and 20th-century doctor: the surgeon, the psychiatrist (or *alienist*) and the general practitioner, doctors who specialise in the body, the mind and the 'whole person' respectively. Compared to the narrow lenses through which the two specialists view their patients, Doyle writes approvingly of the GP Theodore Foster, a man of 'vast experience', with his 'broad humanity', his 'ruddy face and merry eyes'.

William Carlos Williams's *The Use of Force* also recalls an era when house calls, whether by GP or specialist, were much more common than they are today. 'He goes from house to house,' wrote Conan Doyle, 'and his step and his voice are loved and welcomed in each. What could a man ask more than that?' Visiting patients at home gave a paediatrician like Williams an insight into the child's personal and social circumstances. It told him much about who these people really were, and the types of lives they led. On house calls, doctors could learn more about their patients in a few minutes than their hospital colleagues could learn by observing them for several hours, or from all the MRI scans that they carried out on them.

Perhaps unfairly, some of the patient narratives in this collection contrast the holistic role of the generalist with the narrower view of the specialist: the surgeons, oncologists and others that they encounter. Although, as Oliver Sacks's *Rebecca* shows (as does the surgeon Richard Selzer in his moving book *Confessions of a Knife*), specialisation is certainly *not* a bar to a more humane and understanding approach to one's patients.

Today's doctors are an increasingly diverse tribe, and it is increasingly difficult to generalise about them. There are now dozens of different medical specialities and sub-specialities, usually arranged in a hierarchy of income and prestige. In the current medical pecking order, specialists tower over generalists, and surgery and internal medicine are high above family practice. Among the specialists, the psychiatrists, geriatricians and oncologists – and all those others who deal mainly with chronic conditions, where 'care' is as important as 'cure' – tend to have a lower status than the different types of surgeon. Even within surgery there is a hierarchy, with those specialising in parts of the body with the highest symbolic value in our culture – the brain and the heart – having a higher status than, say, those specialising in urology or proctology.

With specialisation can come a narrowing of focus and a clearer boundary between doctor and patient. But in caring for their patients, many of the old-style doctors – whether specialists or generalists – often went way beyond their narrow clinical role, and many of them still do. In this anthology, for example, the neurologist Oliver Sacks visits the handicapped girl Rebecca at home, just after her mother's death; AJ Cronin tries to help the alcoholic David Murray return to normal life by sending him clothes, shoes and money, and finding him a job teaching classics to the son of a friend; Chekhov's Dr Korolyov dines and then stays over with his patient's family, albeit reluctantly; O Henry's Dr Tatum, the old country doctor, cures the hypochondriac's imaginary ills by guile and trickery – taking him on long mountain walks to breathe deeply of the clear country air; and even the remote Dr Lennox, head of the TB sanatorium in Somerset Maugham's story, attends the wedding of his two doomed patients and wishes them well.

Telling bad news

Most clinical encounters between doctors and patients involve some form of struggle (sometimes even a physical one, as in Williams's *The Use of Force* or Bulgakov's *Baptism by Rotation*). A struggle not only between the doctor and the invisible bacteria, viruses or malignant cells that make people ill, but also a struggle of interpretation, of differing explanations, of bad news versus good, hope against despair. A struggle that can leave both parties completely exhausted.

Bad news is always a part of medicine. But telling bad news to patients is never a simple process. Often it is a struggle between the force of two personalities: one trying desperately to negotiate, to reduce or obscure the awfulness of the diagnosis; while on the other side of the doctor's desk, the other one struggles just as hard to maintain their professional demeanour, their mask of emotional detachment. And often, hovering awkwardly in the air in these situations, the unspoken, resentful question: 'Why should *he* survive, and not *me*?'

For Renate Rubinstein, in *Telling the Truth*, revealing *all* the facts to a patient is not always such a good thing. She writes how the one thing she liked about her neurologist was that he *refused* to tell her all the bad news about her multiple sclerosis: 'I meant so much to him,' she writes, '(that) he didn't dare tell me!'

But many other patients would agree, rather, with Samuel Johnson's stern warning to doctors back in the 18th century:

> *I deny the lawfulness of telling a lie to a sick man for fear of alarming him. You have no business with consequences; you are to tell the truth. Besides you may not be sure what effect your telling him that he is in danger may have. It may bring his distemper to a crisis, and that may cure him. Of all lying I have the greatest abhorrence of this, because I believe it has been frequently practised on myself.*

By contrast, Rachel Clark, in her poignant autobiographical piece *Inside Out and Upside Down*, describes the clumsiness of 'Dr Stanton', the ENT surgeon – awkward, embarrassed, evasive, avoiding all eye contact – as he struggles to tell her the awful significance of her particular cancer. Followed then by his registrar, 'Dr Reynolds' – also ill at ease, blurting out the wrong words, at the wrong time. And, in Clive Sinclair's story he, too, tries unsuccessfully to discuss his impending dialysis, and how it will affect his life, with the taciturn surgeon 'Mr T', and his two anonymous assistants, standing silently at the bedside: Dr 'Glasses' and Dr 'Moustache'.

Reading the patient narratives in this book – even O Henry's fictional piece – makes one wonder whether, in modern high-tech medicine, some essence of the patient has almost disappeared, some ancient sense of what it means to be human. In its place, medical attention now focuses on the *body* as a largely physical being, and on the data gathered from it by diagnostic machines. From this process, a new tier of patients has gradually appeared – what I would term *paper patients*: all the printouts of patients' laboratory and other tests, their scan reports and x-ray plates. To some doctors, apparently, these 'patients' seem more attractive than the real thing: certainly less ambiguous, less enquiring and less likely to complain or sue them for malpractice.

This process of abstraction is now increasingly common. In the mid-1980s, when I spent a year as a visiting fellow at a famous medical school in the USA, I was surprised to see – at the first hospital 'Grand Round' I attended – that all the case presentations took place *without* the presence of a single patient. Somehow, over time, the patients had atrophied away, and by now had completely disappeared. Instead, slides and videos of their endoscopies, barium x-rays, blood tests and ultrasound scans were projected on to the screen, in a big auditorium crowded with white-coated doctors and medical students. But not a single patient. The only subjects of discussion were these sparse abstractions of people. In Britain, the process has gone almost as far, although here the patient still usually makes a brief entry to be asked a few perfunctory questions about their illness, before being wheeled quickly out of the room again.

In this high-tech, impersonal setting, the patient's body can become merely a passive battlefield, within which doctors and their wonder drugs wage a deadly war on disease. An invisible battle in which the patient is often reduced to the role of spectator, and the doctors at the bedside into generals and war correspondents – for the war usually takes place invisibly, at the level of cells, hormones or even molecules. This sense of helpless passivity imposed upon them is a feature, I think, of most of the patient narratives included in this book, especially of cancer. The patients find themselves being forced to observe – as if from a great distance – the deadly battle between their own errant cells and the opposing chemical weapons, or death-rays, of the medical army.

In *Travels*, the autobiographical essays of Michael Crichton (creator of *ER* and author of *Jurassic Park*), he describes this impersonal approach as one of the reasons why he eventually left medicine. Based on his own experiences of medical school in the 1960s, and later of a hospital internship, he details his growing disillusionment with the new breed of 'physician-scientist': clever, but insensitive, and often obsessed not with human issues, but with science, especially biochemistry. Unlike his tutors, he:

> didn't think of people as a sack of biochemical reactions that had somehow gone awry. I thought people were complex creatures who sometimes manifested their problems in biochemical terms. But I thought it wiser to deal primarily with the people, not to deal primarily with the biochemistry.

The wounded healer

Franz Kafka's dreamlike and enigmatic parable *A Country Doctor* deals with a different aspect of the doctor–patient relationship. For it hints at a certain deep vulnerability in the medical personality, at the doctor's fear of changing places, of becoming a patient himself. To his horror, the doctor in Kafka's short story finds himself being stripped of his clothes by the family of the patient he is visiting, while in the background the village choir sings 'Strip him naked, then he'll heal us', and being put to bed beside his patient, lying close to the man's bloody, discharging wound.

This story resonates with Oliver Sacks's book *A Leg To Stand On*, which tells how he landed up in a big London hospital after a severe injury to his leg. Here, he finds himself in a *mundus inversus*, an inverted and unfamiliar looking-glass world, in which *he* is the one now lying helplessly in bed, instead of pacing the ward in his white coat.

It seems, though, that some patients actually seem to expect – even to *want* – their healers to be wounded, or at least exhausted, most of the time. Possibly they feel such wounds really *are* necessary for a doctor, in order to develop real empathy with them. For them, those words of the sick man in Kafka's story – 'I came into the world with a fine wound; that's all I have to my name' – should also be true of their own doctors. In *The Healer's Art*, for example, Eric J Cassell describes how often, when he's feeling well and 'fresh as a daisy', his patients tell him how totally *exhausted* he looks, how hard he must work, how little sleep he must be getting. He wonders what they mean by these remarks. Although they are often correct, he suggests that perhaps something else is being said here: that 'fatigue is the real hallmark of the profession, because the struggle of the doctors is with death'. The sign of a good doctor, then, is their very exhaustion: the fatigue of the archetypal hero or heroine, fresh from their daily battle with the cosmic forces of disease and death.

It was only after I studied anthropology that I understood that there *could* be another, very different, way of being a healer. For in many traditional cultures, the healer or shaman (often inaccurately called a 'witch doctor' – for they are neither witch nor doctor) – like the *xaman* in Moacyr Scliar's *The King of Xingu* – embraces their own emotional wound. For the shaman is a 'master of spirits', one who has been possessed by malevolent spirits, but who then masters them in turn. Now, at will, he or she can use their powers to help heal others with the same affliction. Unlike medical doctors, these healers accept being 'ill' (in this case, 'possessed by spirits') as part of their identity and a necessary precondition for being a healer. Many, in fact, *become* shamans in order to heal themselves, so that 'the cure is to become a curer'. Except perhaps for psychoanalysts, the idea of a doctor's own emotional vulnerability playing a positive role in increasing their empathy for patients is a largely taboo subject. Something to be kept at bay by denial, black humour and medical anecdotes.

In truth, though, healing is rarely only one-way, even in Western medicine. The boundaries between doctor and patient are more permeable than they appear. Sometimes it is *patients* who heal doctors – and not the other way round. They do this by appreciation and sympathy and kindness, but also by being healed themselves, thus satisfying their doctor's deep 'need to be needed'.

The cancer specialist Rachel Remen, in her *Kitchen Table Wisdom*, urges doctors to embrace the sense of uncertainty and ambiguity inherent in all clinical practice, and not to avoid it. Furthermore, the good doctor should also embrace their own *vulnerability*, be more open to patients and their humanity, and even – sometimes – be open to being healed *by* them:

> One of the reasons that many physicians feel drained by their work is that they do not know how to make an opening to receive anything from their patients. The way we were trained, receiving is considered unprofessional. The way most of us were raised, receiving is considered a weakness.

Doctors and disillusionment

George Bernard Shaw's remark that 'We have not lost faith, but we have transferred it from God to the medical profession' is probably less true today than it ever was, for public respect for doctors has gradually declined. They live now in an age of increasing malpractice suits, of media campaigns against them and a growing public suspicion – made worse by events such as the thalidomide tragedy and other medical disasters.

These days, people expect much more of their doctors – perhaps far too much. For some people, medicine has become almost a secular religion (with an 'unhealthy lifestyle' replacing 'a sinful life'). For others, the great successes of the antibiotic era, the triumphs of surgery, the rising life expectancy and falling infant mortality rates have all led to a crisis of expectations. And to disillusionment. Renate Rubinstein, for example, expresses a sense of shock that medicine cannot actually *cure* her multiple sclerosis:

> Before I became ill I took it for granted, as do most people, that in our age a good doctor can cure anything, so long as it's not cancer.

The deference of AJ Cronin's day is long gone, too. Today, many of medicine's critics see it as having become more of a business than a noble vocation; a situation where profits have become more important than people and medical care a commodity – available only to those who can afford it. To these critics, the healing of human beings has become a vast, commercial enterprise – often with too-close links to the pharmaceutical industry. Not surprisingly, there is a growing drift towards 'alternative medicine', seen by many as gentler, more personalised, less invasive and somehow more 'natural' than its high-tech opposition.

But the dark side of medical progress has not only been rising costs and drug side effects. It is has also been the development of a new type of doctor alongside the old: less a healer than a technician spouting statistics and scientific theories, someone who converts people into facts and then facts into numbers, and whose attitude to patients is efficient, but strangely impersonal.

Take what happens in hospitals, for example. For all their successes and technical wonders, the picture painted by many patients is often not a sympathetic one. They describe the hospital as a closed, claustrophobic world, where – as in Oliver Sacks's *A Leg To Stand On* – many undergo a process of depersonalisation, a loss of part of their identity. At a time of great anxiety, they find themselves away from family and friends, stripped of their usual clothing, dressed in a uniform of pyjamas or nightgown and lying as a numbered 'case' in a room filled with strangers. Soon, other strangers in white coats will prod and question them, take away their blood and body fluids for analysis, while huge whirring machines will point at, or probe, one part of their body after another.

Doctors can contribute to this sense of alienation. Standing at the bedside, they often speak among themselves in a private dialect, a technical jargon incomprehensible to their patients (like the 'facel-vega' in Sinclair's *My Life as a Pig*). Unlike in the days of Drs Chekhov, Cronin and Maugham, the language of modern medicine has diverged widely from that of patients. In the 1880s, for example, most of the articles in a medical journal like *The Lancet* could be read – and understood – by the educated public. They were anecdotal and subjective, using words and concepts familiar to most non-medical people of the time. By the 1980s, though, they had become opaque, dense, so packed with technical terms that they were virtually incomprehensible to all but the initiated. A situation reflected in some doctor–patient consultations.

The way that young doctors are trained also needs to be looked at anew. I remember as a medical student being sent by one of my tutors to examine 'the spleen, third bed on the left', and then 'that fascinating pair of lungs' or, lying at other end of the ward, 'that absolutely *amazing* mitral valve'. Even today, in many medical schools, students are still trained to begin their understanding of their future patients by first reducing them to their parts – organs, bones, fluids, cells or systems – first in the laboratory and dissecting room, and later in the wards.

Anatomical studies, in particular – although essential to medical training – also involve a violation, a dismantling of the familiar sense of the human body as both unified and complete. Medicine, as Danny Abse puts it, in his poem *X-Ray*, is a form of exploration:

> Some prowl seabeds, some hurtle to a star,
> and, mother, some obsessed turn over every stone
> or open graves to let that starlight in.
> These are men who would open anything.
>
> Harvey, the circulation of the blood,
> and Freud, the circulation of our dreams,
> pried honourably and honoured are
> like all explorers. Men who'd open men.

But human dissection involves a special shift in focus. It is significant that a book of anatomy is still often called an 'atlas'. As if these lavishly illustrated books really were maps of some unknown landscape – not only one hidden away within ourselves, but also somewhere strange, dead, silent and *inhuman*. A land of dead parts, rather than a living unity.

Later, during their clinical studies, one of the student's major tasks will be to reassemble the person, from part to whole, to try to reclaim the elusive sense of the *human*. Much of clinical training can be seen as an exercise in putting a shattered Humpty-Dumpty back together again. Unfortunately, some students will never succeed in doing this. Throughout their medical careers, their patients will remain to them, essentially, as a collection of fragments: a few relevant to their medical treatment, but the rest not.

But whatever the limitations of their training, doctors always carry with them a special, elusive atmosphere. And they always will. After all, a doctor is some-one who has been in the most intimate contact with death and suffering – and yet survived to tell the tale. Who knows more about bodies, their interior and functioning, than their owners ever will. Who is familiar with strange drugs and even stranger diseases. Who is allowed to hurt their patients or make them feel ill – but all in the interests of making them feel better. No wonder patients have such ambivalent, puzzled feelings about their doctors. As Samuel Johnson put it, in his *Life of Mark Akenside*:

> A physician seems to be the mere plaything of fortune; his degree of reputation is for the most part totally casual; they that employ him know not his excellence; they that reject him know not his deficiency.

This anthology, therefore, looks back into medicine's past and offers some clues as to its future – celebrating the *art* of medicine, as much as its science. For in medicine many things are changing now: from the growing AIDS epidemic to the rise of chronic diseases, the increasing costs of medical care to developments in genetic engineering. But in all of this, the true challenge facing a doctor today is exactly the *same* as the one that has faced all previous generations of doctors: how to *heal* – as well as to cure.

Part 1: Doctors

For the doctor there is needed a kindly heart, a gentle touch, the control to keep a confidence, love of children, with the power to make a decision and to accept responsibility.

TB Layton

Physicians of all men are most happy; whatever good success they have the world proclaimeth, and what faults they commit the earth covereth.

Francis Quarles, 1638

If you can't be a king, be a doctor.

Indian proverb

Perhaps the most basic skill of the physician is the ability to have comfort with uncertainty, to recognise with humility the uncertainty inherent in all situations, to be open to the ever-present possibility of the surprising, the mysterious, and even the holy, and to meet people there.

Rachel Naomi Remen

Mikhail Bulgakov

Night. Rain. A tiny clinic in the remote countryside. A difficult birth. A young doctor, recently qualified – but without any experience in obstetrics. These are the elements of Bulgakov's famous story, set in a rural region of Russia, sometime during the First World War. We never learn the name of 'the woman', the one from the village of Dultsevo about to go into labour – only about how her baby lies in an awkward and dangerous position, horizontal in the womb.

For two years after he qualified from medical school in Kiev in 1916, Mikhail Afansyevich Bulgakov practised as a doctor in a remote rural area of south-west Russia, as an alternative to military service. Later, these experiences were to provide him with the material for his fictionalised *A Country Doctor's Notebook*. During his relatively short life, Bulgakov wrote plays, novels, short stories and a biography of Molière. His first book, serialised in 1924, was *Belaya gvardiya* (*The White Guard*). In the 1930s, however, he was accused by the Soviet authorities of 'slandering Soviet reality', and from then on suffered official persecution. For many years they prevented his books from being published in Russia, and his was a life of frustration and unhappiness. His most famous novel, *The Master and Margarita*, was only published posthumously.

In Bulgakov's story, the difficult labour and birth is also that of the narrator himself. He becomes, for the first time, a *real* doctor – baptised in blood and sweat – born from theory into practice, from book learning into the realities of medical life.

Baptism by Rotation

by Mikhail Bulgakov

As time passed in my country hospital, I gradually got used to the new way of life.

They were braking flax in the villages as they had always done, the roads were still impassable, and no more than five patients came to my daily surgery. My evenings were entirely free, and I spent them sorting out the library, reading surgical manuals and spending long hours drinking tea alone with the gently humming samovar.

For whole days and nights it poured with rain, the drops pounded unceasingly on the roof and the water cascaded past my window, swirling along the gutter and into a tub. Outside was slush, darkness and fog, through which the windows of the *feldsher*'s house and the kerosene lantern over the gateway were no more than faint, blurred patches of light.

On one such evening I was sitting in my study with an atlas of topographical anatomy. The absolute silence was only disturbed by the occasional gnawing of mice behind the sideboard in the dining-room.

I read until my eyelids grew so heavy that they began to stick together. Finally I yawned, put the atlas aside and decided to go to bed. I stretched in pleasant anticipation of sleeping soundly to the accompaniment of the noisy pounding of the rain, then went across to my bedroom, undressed and lay down.

No sooner had my head touched the pillow than there swam hazily before me the face of Anna Prokhorova, a girl of seventeen from the village of Toropovo. She had needed a tooth extracting. Demyan Lukich, the *feldsher*, floated silently past holding a gleaming pair of pincers. Remembering how he always said 'suchlike' instead of 'such' because he was fond of a high-falutin' style, I smiled and fell asleep.

About half an hour later, however, I suddenly woke up as though I had been pinched, sat up, stared fearfully into the darkness and listened.

Someone was drumming loudly and insistently on the outer door and I immediately sensed that those knocks boded no good.

Then came a knock on the door of my quarters.

The noise stopped, there was a grating of bolts, the sound of the cook talking, an indistinct voice in reply, then someone came creaking up the stairs, passed quietly through the study and knocked on my bedroom door.

'Who is it?'

'It's me,' came the reply in a respectful whisper. 'Me, Aksinya, the nurse.'

'What's the matter?'

'Anna Nikolaevna has sent for you. They want you to come to the hospital as quickly as possible.'

'What's happened?' I asked, feeling my heart literally miss a beat.

'A woman has been brought in from Dultsevo. She's having a difficult labour.'

'Here we go!' I thought to myself, quite unable to get my feet into my slippers. 'Hell, the matches won't light. Ah well, it had to happen sooner or later. You can't expect to get nothing but cases of laryngitis or abdominal catarrh all your life.'

'All right, go and tell them I'm coming at once!' I shouted as I got out of bed. Aksinya's footsteps shuffled away from the door and the bolt grated again. Sleep vanished in a moment. Hurriedly, with shaking fingers, I lit the lamp and began dressing. Half past eleven . . . What could be wrong with this woman who was having a difficult birth? Malpresentation? Narrow pelvis? Or perhaps something worse. I might even have to use forceps. Should I send her straight into town? Out of the question! A fine doctor he is, they'll all say. In any case, I have no right to do that. No, I really must do it myself. But do what? God alone knows. It would be disastrous if I lost my head – I might disgrace myself in front of the midwives. Anyway, I must have a look first; no point in getting worried prematurely . . .

I dressed, threw an overcoat over my shoulders, and hoping that all would be well, ran to the hospital through the rain across the creaking duckboards. At the entrance I could see a cart in the semi-darkness, the horse pawing at the rotten boards under its hooves.

'Did you bring the woman in labour?' I asked the figure lurking by the horse.

'Yes, that's right . . . we did, sir,' a woman's voice replied dolefully.

Despite the hour, the hospital was alive and bustling. A flickering pressure-lamp was burning in the surgery. In the little passage leading to the delivery room Aksinya slipped past me carrying a basin. A faint moan came through the door and died away again. I opened the door and went into the delivery room. The small, whitewashed room was brightly lit by a lamp in the ceiling. On a bed alongside the operating table, covered with a blanket up to her chin, lay a young woman. Her face was contorted in a grimace of pain and wet strands of hair were sticking to her forehead. Holding a large thermometer, Anna Nikolaevna was preparing a solution in a graduated jug, while Pelagea Ivanovna was getting clean sheets out of the cupboard. The *feldsher* was leaning against the wall in a Napoleonic pose. Seeing me, they all jerked into life. The pregnant woman opened her eyes, wrung her hands and renewed her pathetic, long drawn-out groaning.

'Well now, what seems to be the trouble?' I asked, sounding confident.

'Transverse lie,' Anna Nikolaevna answered promptly as she went on pouring water into the solution.

'I see-ee,' I drawled, and added, frowning: 'Well, let's have a look . . .'

'Aksinya! Wash the doctor's hands!' snapped Anna Nikolaevna. Her expression was solemn and serious.

As the water flowed, rinsing away the lather from my hands, reddened from scrubbing, I asked Anna Nikolaevna a few trivial questions, such as when the woman had been brought in, where she was from . . . Pelagea Ivanovna's hand turned back the blanket, I sat down on the edge of the bed and began gently feeling the swollen belly. The woman groaned, stretched, dug her fingers into her flesh and crumpled the sheet.

'There, there, relax . . . it won't take long,' I said as I carefully put my hands to the hot, dry, distended skin.

The fact was that once the experienced Anna Nikolaevna had told me what was wrong, this examination was quite pointless. I could examine the woman as much as I liked, but I would not find out any more than Anna Nikolaevna knew already. Her diagnosis was, of course, correct: transverse lie. It was obvious. Well, what next?

Frowning, I continued palpating the belly on all sides and glanced sidelong at the midwives' faces. Both were watching with intense concentration and their looks registered approval of what I was doing. But although my movements were confident and correct, I did my best to conceal my unease as thoroughly as possible.

'Very well,' I said with a sigh, standing up from the bed, as there was nothing more to be seen from an external examination. 'Let's examine her internally.'

Another look of approval from Anna Nikolaevna.

'Aksinya!'

More water flowed.

'Oh, if only I could consult Döderlein now!' I thought miserably as I soaped my hands. Alas, this was quite impossible. In any case, how could Döderlein help me at a moment like this? I washed off the thick lather and painted my fingers with iodine. A clean sheet rustled in Pelagea Ivanovna's hands and, bending down over the expectant mother, I began cautiously and timidly to carry out an internal examination. Into my mind came an involuntary recollection of the operating theatre in the maternity hospital. Gleaming electric lights in frosted-glass globes, a shining tiled floor, taps and instruments a-glitter everywhere. A junior registrar in a snow-white coat is manipulating the woman, surrounded by three intern assistants, probationers, and a crowd of students doing their practicals. Everything bright, well ordered and safe.

And there was I, all on my own, with a woman in agony on my hands and I was responsible for her. I had no idea, however, what I was supposed to do to help her, because I had seen childbirth at close quarters only twice in my life in a hospital, and both occasions were completely normal. The fact that I was conducting an examination was of no value to me or to the woman; I understood absolutely nothing and could feel nothing of what was inside her.

It was time to make some sort of decision.

'Transverse lie . . . since it's a transverse lie I must . . . I must . . . '

'Turn it round by the foot,' muttered Anna Nikolaevna as though thinking aloud, unable to restrain herself.

An older, more experienced doctor would have looked askance at her for butting in, but I am not the kind to take offence.

'Yes,' I concurred gravely, 'a podalic version.'

The pages of Döderlein flickered before my eyes. Internal method . . . Combined method . . . External method . . . Page after page, covered in illustrations. A pelvis; twisted, crushed babies with enormous heads . . . a little dangling arm with a loop on it.

Indeed I had read it not long ago and had underlined it, soaking up every word, mentally picturing the interrelationship of every part of the whole and every method. And as I read it I imagined that the entire text was being imprinted on my brain for ever.

Yet now only one sentence of it floated back into my memory:

A transverse lie is a wholly unfavourable position.

Too true. Wholly unfavourable both for the woman and for a doctor who only qualified six months ago.

'Very well, we'll do it,' I said as I stood up.

Anna Nikolaevna's expression came to life.

'Demyan Lukich,' she turned to the *feldsher*, 'get the chloroform ready.'

It was a good thing that she had said so, because I was still not certain whether the operation was supposed to be done under anaesthesia or not! Of course, under anaesthesia – how else?

Still, I must have a look at Döderlein . . .

As I washed my hands I said: 'All right, then . . . prepare her for anaesthesia and make her comfortable. I'll be back in a moment; I must just go to my room and fetch some cigarettes.'

'Very good, doctor, we'll be ready by the time you come back,' replied Anna Nikolaevna.

I dried my hands, the nurse threw my coat over my shoulders and without putting my arms into the sleeves I set off for home at a run.

In my study I lit the lamp and, forgetting to take off my cap, rushed straight to the bookcase.

There it was – Döderlein's *Operative Obstetrics*. I began hastily to leaf through the glossy pages.

. . . version is always a dangerous operation for the mother . . .

A cold shiver ran down my spine.

The chief danger lies in the possibility of a spontaneous rupture of the uterus . . .

Spon-tan-e-ous . . .

If in introducing his hand into the uterus the obstetrician encounters any hindrances to penetrating to the foot, whether from lack of space or as a result of a contraction of the uterine wall, he should refrain from further attempts to carry out the version . . .

Good. Provided I am able, by some miracle, to recognise these 'hindrances' and I refrain from 'further attempts', what, might I ask, am I then supposed to do with an anaesthetised woman from the village of Dultsevo?

Further:

It is absolutely impermissible to attempt to reach the feet by penetrating behind the back of the foetus . . .

Noted.

It must be regarded as erroneous to grasp the upper leg, as doing so may easily result in the foetus being revolved too far; this can cause the foetus to suffer a severe blow, which can have the most deplorable consequences . . .

'Deplorable consequences.' Rather a vague phrase, but how sinister. What if the husband of the woman from Dultsevo is left a widower? I wiped the sweat from my brow, rallied my strength and disregarded all the terrible things that could go wrong, trying only to remember the absolute essentials: what I had to do, where and how to put my hands. But as I ran my eye over the lines of black print, I kept encountering new horrors. They leaped out at me from the page.

. . . in view of the extreme danger of rupture . . .

. . . the internal and combined methods must be classified as among the most dangerous obstetric operations to which a mother can be subjected . . .

And as a grand finale:

. . . with every hour of delay the danger increases . . .

That was enough. My reading had borne fruit: my head was in a complete muddle. For a moment I was convinced that I understood nothing, and above all that I had no idea what sort of version I was going to perform: combined, bi-polar, internal, external . . .

I abandoned Döderlein and sank into an armchair, struggling to reduce my random thoughts to order. Then I glanced at my watch. Hell! I had already spent twenty minutes in my room, and they were waiting for me.

. . . with every hour of delay . . .

Hours are made up of minutes, and at times like this the minutes fly past at insane speed. I threw Döderlein aside and ran back to the hospital.

Everything there was ready. The *feldsher* was standing over a little table preparing the anaesthetic mask and the chloroform bottle. The expectant mother already lay on the operating table. Her ceaseless moans could be heard all over the hospital.

'There now, be brave,' Pelagea Ivanovna muttered consolingly as she bent over the woman, 'the doctor will help you in a moment.'

'Oh, no! I haven't the strength . . . No . . . I can't stand it!'

'Don't be afraid,' whispered the midwife. 'You'll stand it. We'll just give you something to sniff, and then you won't feel anything.'

Water gushed noisily from the taps as Anna Nikolaevna and I began washing and scrubbing our arms bared to the elbow. Against a background of groans and screams Anna Nikolaevna described to me how my predecessor, an experienced surgeon, had performed versions. I listened avidly to her, trying not to miss a single word. Those ten minutes told me more than everything I had read on obstetrics for my qualifying exams, in which I had actually passed the obstetrics paper 'with distinction'. From her brief remarks, unfinished sentences and passing hints I learned the essentials which are not to be found in any textbooks. And by the time I had begun to dry the perfect whiteness and cleanliness of my hands with sterile gauze, I was seized with confidence and a firm and absolutely definite plan had formed in my mind. There was simply no need to bother any longer over whether it was to be a combined or bi-polar version.

None of these learned words meant anything at that moment. Only one thing mattered: I had to put one hand inside, assist the version with the other hand from outside and without relying on books but on common sense, without which no doctor is any good, carefully but firmly bring one foot downwards and pull the baby after it.

I had to be calm and cautious yet at the same time utterly decisive and unfaltering.

'Right, off you go,' I instructed the *feldsher* as I began painting my fingers with iodine.

At once Pelagea Ivanovna folded the woman's arms and the *feldsher* clamped the mask over her agonised face. Chloroform slowly began to drip out of the dark yellow glass bottle, and the room started to fill with the sweet, nauseous odour. The expressions of the *feldsher* and midwives hardened with concentration, as though inspired . . .

'Haaa! Ah!' The woman suddenly shrieked. For a few seconds she writhed convulsively, trying to force away the mask.

'Hold her!'

Pelagea Ivanovna seized her by the arms and lay across her chest. The woman cried out a few more times, jerking her face away from the mask. Her movements slowed down, although she mumbled dully:

'Oh . . . let me go . . . ah . . .'

She grew weaker and weaker. The white room was silent. The translucent drops continued to drip, drip, drip on to the white gauze.

'Pulse, Pelagea Ivanovna?'

'Firm.'

Pelagea Ivanovna raised the woman's arm and let it drop: as lifeless as a leather thong, it flopped on to the sheet. Removing the mask, the *feldsher* examined the pupil of her eye.

'She's asleep.'

A pool of blood. My arms covered in blood up to the elbows. Bloodstains on the sheets. Red clots and lumps of gauze. Pelagea Ivanovna shaking and slapping the baby, Aksinya rattling buckets as she poured water into basins.

The baby was dipped alternately into cold and hot water. He did not make a sound, his head flopping lifelessly from side to side as though on a thread. Then suddenly there came a noise somewhere between a squeak and a sigh, followed by the first weak, hoarse cry.

'He's alive . . . alive . . .' mumbled Pelagea Ivanovna as she laid the baby on a pillow.

And the mother was alive. Fortunately nothing had gone wrong. I felt her pulse. Yes, it was firm and steady; the *feldsher* gently shook her by the shoulder as he said:

'Wake up now, my dear.'

The bloodstained sheets were thrown aside and the mother hastily covered with a clean one before the *feldsher* and Aksinya wheeled her away to the ward. The swaddled baby was borne away on his pillow, the brown, wrinkled little face staring out from its white wrapping as he cried ceaselessly in a thin, pathetic whimper.

Water gushing from the taps of the sluice. Anna Nikolaevna coughed as she dragged hungrily at a cigarette.

'You did the version well, doctor. You seemed very confident.'

Scrubbing furiously at my hands, I glanced sidelong at her: was she being sarcastic? But no, her expression was a sincere one of pride and satisfaction. My heart was brimming with joy. I glanced round at the white and bloodstained disorder, at the red water in the basin and felt that I had won. But somewhere deep down there wriggled a worm of doubt.

'Let's wait and see what happens now,' I said.

Anna Nikolaevna turned to look at me in astonishment.

'What can happen? Everything's all right.'

I mumbled something vague in reply. What I had meant to say was to wonder whether the mother was really safe and sound, whether I might not have done her some harm during the operation . . . the thought nagged dully at my mind. My knowledge of obstetrics was so vague, so fragmentary and bookish. What about a rupture? How would it show? And when would it show – now or, perhaps, later? Better not talk about that.

'Well, almost anything,' I said. 'The possibility of infection cannot be ruled out,' I added, repeating the first sentence from some textbook that came into my mind.

'Oh, tha-at,' Anna Nikolaevna drawled complacently. 'Well, with luck nothing of that sort will happen. How could it, anyway? Everything here is clean and sterile.'

It was after one o'clock when I went back to my room. In a pool of light on the desk in my study lay Döderlein open at the page headed 'Dangers of Version'. For another hour after that, sipping my cooling tea, I sat over it, turning the pages. And an interesting thing happened: all the previously obscure passages became entirely comprehensible, as though they had been flooded with light; and there, at night, under the lamplight in the depth of the countryside I realised what real knowledge was.

'One can gain a lot of experience in a country practice,' I thought as I fell asleep, 'but even so one must go on and on reading, reading . . . more and more . . .'

Franz Kafka

I came into the world with a fine wound: that's all I have to my name,

is the emblematic sentence of this haunting and mysterious story – a story that has all the elements of a dream, or rather a nightmare.

Like Anton Chekhov's *Ward Five*, *A Country Doctor* is all about the fragile psychological membrane that separates doctor and patient – and how, under some circumstance, it can easily disappear, so that one dissolves into the other.

Franz Kafka – one of the most original writers of the 20th century – was born in Prague in 1883 and, after studying literature and medicine for a short time, eventually obtained his doctorate in law from Prague University. Later, he worked as a minor official in an insurance company. Although a Czech, his novels, short stories and parables were all written in German. Kafka died of tuberculosis in 1924, and some of his most famous books were published posthumously, including *The Trial* (1925), *The Castle* (1926), *America* (1927) and *The Great Wall of China* (1931). He has given the word 'Kafkaesque' to the English language – a word that conveys a dreamlike atmosphere of ill-defined terror and shadowy paranoia.

Ein Landartz (A Country Doctor) was first published in 1919, as part of a collection of 14 short stories. It is believed that the character of the doctor was based on Kafka's favourite uncle Siegfried Lowy (1867–1942), himself a country doctor in Moravia.

A Country Doctor

by Franz Kafka

I was at my wit's end: an urgent journey lay ahead of me; a seriously ill patient was expecting me in a village ten miles off; a dense snowstorm filled the wide space between him and me; I had a trap, a light trap with big wheels, just right for our country roads; muffled in furs, instrument bag in my hand, I stood ready and waiting in the courtyard; but not a horse was to be had, not a horse. My own horse had died in the night, worn out by the grind of this icy winter; my servant girl was now running round the village to get the loan of a horse; but it was hopeless, I knew it, and there I stood aimlessly, more and more snowed under, more and more unable to move. The girl appeared in the gateway, alone, and swung the lantern; but who lends his horse at a time like this for a journey like that? I strode across the courtyard again; I could think of no alternative; upset, I absent-mindedly gave a kick to the ramshackle door of the ancient unused pig-sty. It flew open and flapped to and fro on its hinges. A horselike warmth and stench came out to meet me. A dim stable lantern was swinging inside on a rope. A man, squatting down in that low hovel, showed his face, frank and blue-eyed. 'Shall I yoke up?' he asked, crawling out on all fours. I didn't know what to say and merely bent down to see what else was in the shed. The servant girl was standing beside me. 'You just don't know what you're going to stumble across in your own house' she said, and we both laughed. 'Hey Brother, hey Sister!' the stable boy called, and two horses, huge beasts with strong flanks, legs flush against the torso, shapely heads bent like camels, only by powerful contortions of their hindquarters squeezed out one behind the other through the keyhole which they filled entirely. At once they stood there, long-legged, their bodies thick clouds of steam. 'Give him a hand', I said, and the girl promptly hurried over to help the stable boy with the harnessing. Hardly was she beside him when he grabbed hold of her and pressed his face against hers. She screamed and fled back to me; the imprint of two rows of teeth stood out red on her cheek. 'You beast', I yelled in fury, 'do you want a whipping?', but at the same time realised he was a stranger; that I didn't know where he'd come from, and that he was volunteering to help me out when everyone else had turned a deaf ear. As if he'd read my mind, he took no offence at my threat, and instead simply turned towards me once more while he worked with the horses. 'Get in', he said, and sure enough: everything was ready. I'd never ridden, I thought, with such a splendid pair of horses, and I climbed in cheerfully. 'But I'll take the reins', I said, 'You don't know the way.' 'Sure', he said, 'I'm not coming with you anyway, I'm staying with Rose.' 'No', shrieked Rose and rushed into the house, knowing in her bones that her fate couldn't be averted; I heard the door-chain clatter as she put it up; I heard the key scrape in the lock; I also saw how she put the lights out, first in the corridor and then from room to room, to prevent herself from being found. 'You're coming with me', I said to the stable boy, 'or I'm not going at all, urgent though the journey is. I wouldn't even think of paying for it by handing you the girl.' 'Gee up!', he said; clapped his hands; the trap sprang off like a log in a rapid; I could just hear the door of my house split and burst under the stable boy's assault, and then I was blinded and deafened by a roaring noise that buffeted all my senses. But that too for only a moment, since already I was there as if my patient's yard had opened out just in front of my own gate; the horses were standing quietly; it had stopped snowing; moonlight all around; my patient's parents hurrying out of the house; his sister behind them; they almost lifted me out of the carriage; I couldn't catch anything of their confused talking all at once; in the sick-room the air was hardly fit to breath; the stove was unattended and smoking away; I thought to heave open the window; but first I wanted to see my patient. Gaunt, no fever, not cold, not warm, his eyes vacant, the young man hauled himself up shirtless from under his eiderdown, clasped my neck, and whispered in my ear: 'Doctor, let me die.' I glanced around; nobody had heard it; the parents stood stooped and silent, awaiting my verdict; the sister had set a chair for my doctor's bag. I opened the bag and rummaged through my instruments; the young man kept leaning out of bed to grasp me, and remind me of his plea; I picked up a pair of forceps, examined them in the candle light and put them down again. 'Yes', I thought blasphemously, 'in cases like this the gods help out, send the missing horse, couple it with another because of the urgency, and then to crown it all donate a stable boy –' And only then did I think of Rose again; what was I to do, how could I rescue her, how could I pull her out from under that stable boy, ten miles away from her, my carriage drawn by ungovernable horses? These horses, they'd somehow slipped loose of the reins; pushed open the windows, I don't know how, from outside; each stuck a head in through a window and undeterred by the family's commotion, ogled the patient. 'I'll go back straightaway', I thought, as if the horses were summoning me for the trip, but I allowed the sister, who thought me dazed by the heat, to relieve me of my fur coat. A glass of rum was laid out for me, the old man clapped me on the shoulder, his familiarity justified by the offer of his prized rum. I shook my head; in the immediate confines of the old man's thinking I felt ill; only for that reason did I decline the drink. The mother stood by the bed and enticed me towards it; I yielded and while one of the horses brayed loudly at the ceiling laid my head on the young man's chest which trembled under my wet beard. It confirmed what I already knew: the young man was healthy, a few circulatory problems, saturated with coffee by the solicitous mother, but healthy and best bundled out of bed with a good shove. I'm no world reformer, so I let him lie. I'm the district doctor and do my duty as far as possible, to the brink of overdoing it. Badly paid, but I give what I have, ready to help the poor. I still have to look after Rose, and then the young man might be right and I too about to die. What was I doing here in this endless winter! My horse was dead, and nobody in the village would lend me another. I'd had to get my team out of the pig-sty; if they hadn't happened to be horses, I would have been travelling with pigs. That's how it was. And I nodded to the family. They knew nothing about it, and had they known, wouldn't have believed it. Writing prescriptions is easy, but coming to an understanding with people is hard. So, that should have been that, my visit ended, called out unnecessarily once again: I was used to it, the whole district tortured me with my night-bell; but that I'd had to surrender Rose this time too, the lovely girl who'd lived in my house for years without my hardly noticing – this sacrifice was too much, and I somehow had to make sense of it in my head by splitting hairs, so as not to fly straight for this family which, with the best will in the world, couldn't give Rose back to me. But when I shut my bag and beckoned for my fur coat, the family standing together, the father sniffing at the glass of rum in his hand, the mother in all likelihood disappointed by me – but what do people expect? – biting her lips, tears in her eyes, the sister brandishing a blood-drenched handkerchief, I was somehow ready to concede the young man might possibly be ill after all. I approached him, he greeted me with a smile as if I were bringing him the most nutritious broth – ah, now both the horses were neighing; the noise must surely have been ordered from above to facilitate my examination – and this time I discovered the young man was indeed ill. In his right side, near the hip, a wound had opened, as big as my palm. Rose-red, in variegated hues, dark at its base and lighter at the margins, slightly granulated, with irregular pockets of blood, open like a mine to the day above. So it looked from the distance. On closer inspection, there was an added complication. Who could look at that without whistling under his breath? Worms, as long and broad as my little finger, themselves rose-red and blood-spattered besides, squirmed up from their fastness within the wound towards the light, with small white heads and lots of tiny legs. Poor young man, there's no helping you. I've discovered your great wound; this blossom in your flank is dragging you down. The family was pleased, watched me busying myself; sister told mother, mother father, father a few guests who were coming in on tiptoe through the moonlight from the open door, arms outstretched to hold their balance. 'Will you save me?' sobbed the young man in a whisper, quite dazzled by the life in his wound. That's what people are like in this region. Always expecting the impossible from the doctor. They've lost their old beliefs; the cleric sits at home and unpicks his vestments, one after another; but the doctor is expected to be able to do everything with his gentle surgeon's hand. Well, as they wish it: I didn't thrust my services on them; should they misuse me for sacred purposes, I wouldn't stand in their way with that either; how could I expect anything better, old country doctor that I am, robbed of my servant girl! And so they came, the family and the village elders, and stripped me of my clothes; a school choir with the teacher at its head stood in front of the house and sang these words to an extremely simple tune:

> Strip him naked, then he'll heal us
> And should he fail to, kill him quick!
> Only a mediciner, only a mediciner.

Then my clothes were off and I looked at the people quietly, fingers in my beard and my head to one side. I was calm and collected and a match for the situation, and I stayed like that, although it wouldn't help me, for now they took me by the head and feet and carried me to the bed. They laid me beside the wall, on the side of the wound. Then they all left the room; the door was shut; the singing ceased; clouds covered the moon; the bedding was warm around me; the horses' heads flickered like shadows in the window-frames. 'Do you know', said a voice in my ear, 'I don't have much confidence in you. After all, you were only blown in here, you didn't come on your own two feet. Instead of helping, you're cramping my death bed. I'd like best to scratch your eyes out.' 'You're right', I said, 'it's a disgrace. But then I'm just a doctor. What was I to do? Believe me, it's none too easy for me either.' 'Am I supposed to accept your apology? Oh, I have to: I always have to put up with things. I came into the world with a fine wound; that's all I have to my name.' 'Young friend,' I said, 'your error is this: you lack perspective. I've been in all the sick-rooms, far and wide, and I tell you: your wound isn't so bad. Done in a tight jam with two blows of the axe. Many a person offers up his side and hardly hears the axe in the forest, much less that it's nearing him.' 'Is that really so, or are you deluding me in my fever?' 'That's the truth, take the word of honour of a medical officer.' And he took it and lay quiet. But now it was time for me to think of saving myself. The horses were still standing faithfully in their place. Clothes, fur coat and bag were quickly grabbed; I didn't want to waste time dressing; if the horses raced home the way they'd come, I'd only be leaping in a manner of speaking from this bed into my own. Obediently a horse backed away from the window; I threw my bundle into the carriage; the fur coat flew too far and snagged on a hook only by the sleeve. Good enough. I swung myself on the horse. The reins loosely dragging, one horse barely coupled to the other, the carriage lurching behind, the fur coat straggling in the snow. 'Gee up!' I said, but it was anything but brisk; like old men we went slowly through the snowy wastes; a long time resounding behind us the children's latest, if mistaken song:

Now be cheerful, all you patients,
Doctor's laid in bed beside you!

At this rate I'll never reach home; my flourishing practice has gone to the wall; my successor is robbing me, but in vain, since he can't replace me; the loathsome stable boy is running riot in my house; Rose is his victim; I can't bear to think about it. Naked, exposed to the frost of this most unfortunate of times, with an earthly carriage, unearthly horses, old vagabond that I am. My fur coat's hanging at the back of the carriage, but I can't reach it, and not one of my agile pack of patients lifts a finger. Betrayed! Betrayed! Respond to a false alarm on the night-bell – and it can't be made good, ever again.

Arthur Conan Doyle

Twenty coffee cups, a dozen liqueur glasses, and a solid bank of blue smoke which swirls slowly along the high, gilded ceiling.

The stage is set for the three doctors to swap their medical stories. Three wise medical men: the psychiatrist, the general practitioner and the surgeon.

Arthur Conan Doyle – creator of Sherlock Holmes – was born in Scotland, and qualified as a doctor at the University of Edinburgh in 1881. He described medicine as 'a noble, generous, kindly profession', and at various times worked as a general physician, a ship's doctor, an eye specialist and the director of a military hospital, but in 1890 he gave up medicine to write full time. The character of Sherlock Holmes was said to be based on Dr Joseph Bell, a fine diagnostician, and one of his lecturers at Edinburgh. In the Holmes stories, Conan Doyle splits the doctor from the diagnostician: Watson, the retired physician, kind, loyal, open-hearted and dull (doomed only to record his master's more interesting 'case histories'), from Holmes, the emotionally detached scientist, author of learned treatises and keen observer of human foibles. A split that, in a way, presages a wider split within the medical profession. But it is the way that Holmes combines his scientific approach with another side of his personality – his intuition, fine sensitivity and creative way of thinking – that is his true genius. Holmes is the ultimate diagnostician, detecting the pattern of clues behind the mask of appearances, the meaning hidden behind the mystery.

The following story, *A Medical Document*, is taken from Conan Doyle's book of short stories, *Tales of Adventure and Medical Life*, first published in 1922. Ten of the stories in the book have a medical background, and it is likely that all, or some of them, drew on his own medical experiences.

A Medical Document

by Arthur Conan Doyle

Medical men are, as a class, very much too busy to take stock of singular situations or dramatic events. Thus it happens that the ablest chronicler of their experiences in our literature was a lawyer. A life spent in watching over death-beds – or over birth-beds which are infinitely more trying – takes something from a man's sense of proportion, as constant strong waters might corrupt his palate. The over-stimulated nerve ceases to respond. Ask the surgeon for his best experiences and he may reply that he has seen little that is remarkable, or break away into the technical. But catch him some night when the fire has spurted up and his pipe is reeking, with a few of his brother practitioners for company and an artful question or allusion to set him going. Then you will get some raw, green facts new plucked from the tree of life.

It is after one of the quarterly dinners of the Midland Branch of the British Medical Association. Twenty coffee cups, a dozen liqueur glasses, and a solid bank of blue smoke which swirls slowly along the high, gilded ceiling gives a hint of a successful gathering. But the members have shredded off to their homes. The line of heavy, bulge-pocketed overcoats and of stethoscope-bearing top hats is gone from the hotel corridor. Round the fire in the sitting-room three medicos are still lingering, however, all smoking and arguing, while a fourth, who is a mere layman and young at that, sits back at the table. Under cover of an open journal he is writing furiously with a stylographic pen, asking a question in an innocent voice from time to time and so flickering up the conversation whenever it shows a tendency to wane.

The three men are all of that staid middle age which begins early and lasts late in the profession. They are none of them famous, yet each is of good repute, and a fair type of his particular branch. The portly man with the authoritative manner and the white, vitriol splash upon his cheek is Charley Manson, chief of the Wormley Asylum, and author of the brilliant monograph, 'Obscure Nervous Lesions in the Unmarried'. He always wears his collar high like that, since the half-successful attempt of a student of

Revelations to cut his throat with a splinter of glass. The second, with the ruddy face and the merry brown eyes, is a general practitioner, a man of vast experience, who, with his three assistants and his five horses, takes twenty-five hundred a year in half-crown visits and shilling consultations out of the poorest quarter of a great city. That cheery face of Theodore Foster is seen at the side of a hundred sick-beds a day, and if he has one-third more names on his visiting list than in his cash-book he always promises himself that he will get level some day when a millionaire with a chronic complaint – the ideal combination – shall seek his services. The third, sitting on the right with his dress-shoes shining on the top of the fender, is Hargrave, the rising surgeon. His face has none of the broad humanity of Theodore Foster's, the eye is stern and critical, the mouth straight and severe, but there is strength and decision in every line of it, and it is nerve rather than sympathy which the patient demands when he is bad enough to come to Hargrave's door. He calls himself a jawman, 'a mere jawman', as he modestly puts it, but in point of fact he is too young and too poor to confine himself to a speciality, and there is nothing surgical which Hargrave has not the skill and the audacity to do.

'Before, after, and during,' murmurs the general practitioner in answer to some interpolation of the outsider's. 'I assure you, Manson, one sees all sorts of evanescent forms of madness.'

'Ah, puerperal!' throws in the other, knocking the curved, grey ash from his cigar. 'But you had some case in your mind, Foster.'

'Well, there was one only last week which was new to me. I had been engaged by some people of the name of Silcoe. When the trouble came round I went myself, for they would not hear of an assistant. The husband, who was a policeman, was sitting at the head of the bed on the farther side. "This won't do," said I. "Oh yes, doctor, it must do," said she. "It's quite irregular, and he must go," said I. "It's that or nothing," said she. "I won't open my mouth or stir a finger the whole night," said he. So it ended by my allowing him to remain, and there he sat for eight hours on end. She was very good over the matter, but every now and again *he* would fetch a hollow groan, and I noticed that he held his right hand just under the sheet all the time, where I had no doubt that it was clasped by her left. When it was all happily over, I looked at him and his face was the colour of this cigar ash, and his head had dropped on to the edge of the pillow. Of course I thought he had fainted with emotion, and I was just telling myself what I thought of myself for having been such a fool as to let him stay there, when suddenly I saw that the sheet over his hand was all soaked with blood; I whisked it down, and there was the fellow's wrist half cut through. The woman had one bracelet of a policeman's handcuff over her left wrist and the other round his right one. When she had been in pain she had twisted with all her strength and the iron had fairly eaten into the bone of the man's arm. "Aye, doctor," said she, when she saw I had noticed it. "He's got to take his share as well as me. Turn and turn," said she.'

'Don't you find it a very wearing branch of the profession?' asks Foster after a pause.

'My dear fellow, it was the fear of it that drove me into lunacy work.'

'Aye, and it has driven men into asylums who never found their way on to the medical staff. I was a very shy fellow myself as a student, and I know what it means.'

'No joke that in general practice,' says the alienist.

'Well, you hear men talk about it as though it were, but I tell you it's much nearer tragedy. Take some poor, raw, young fellow who has just put up his plate in a strange town. He has found it a trial all his life, perhaps, to talk to a woman about lawn tennis and church services. When a young man *is* shy he is shyer than any girl. Then down comes an anxious mother and consults him upon the most intimate family matters. "I shall never go to that doctor again," says she afterwards. "His manner is so stiff and unsympathetic." Unsympathetic! Why, the poor lad was struck dumb and paralysed. I have known general practitioners who were so shy that they could not bring themselves to ask the way in the street. Fancy what sensitive men like that must endure before they get broken into medical practice. And then they know that nothing is so catching as shyness, and that if they do not keep a face of stone, their patient will be covered with confusion. And so they keep their face of stone, and earn the reputation perhaps of having a heart to correspond. I suppose nothing would shake *your* nerve, Manson.'

'Well, when a man lives year in year out among a thousand lunatics, with a fair sprinkling of homicidals among them, one's nerves either get set or shattered. Mine are all right so far.'

'I was frightened once,' says the surgeon. 'It was when I was doing dispensary work. One night I had a call from some very poor people, and gathered from the few words they said that their child was ill. When I entered the room I saw a small cradle in the corner. Raising the lamp I walked over and putting back the curtains I looked down at the baby. I tell you it was sheer Providence that I didn't drop that lamp and set the whole place alight. The head on the pillow turned, and I saw a face looking up at me which seemed to me to have more malignancy and wickedness than ever I had dreamed of in a nightmare. It was the flush of red over the cheek-bones, and the brooding eyes full of loathing of me, and of everything else, that impressed me. I'll never forget my start as, instead of the chubby face of an infant, my eyes fell upon this creature. I took the mother into the next room. "What is it?" I asked. "A girl of sixteen," said she, and then throwing up her arms, "Oh, pray God she may be taken!" The poor thing, though she spent her life in this little cradle, had great, long, thin limbs which she curled up under her. I lost sight of the case and don't know what became of it, but I'll never forget the look in her eyes.'

'That's creepy,' says Doctor Foster. 'But I think one of my experiences would run it close. Shortly after I put up my plate I had a visit from a little hunchbacked woman, who wished me to come and attend to her sister in her trouble.

When I reached the house, which was a very poor one, I found two other little hunch-backed women, exactly like the first, waiting for me in the sitting-room. Not one of them said a word, but my companion took the lamp and walked upstairs with her two sisters behind her, and me bringing up the rear. I can see those three queer shadows cast by the lamp upon the wall as clearly as I can see that tobacco pouch. In the room above was the fourth sister, a remarkably beautiful girl in evident need of my assistance. There was no wedding-ring upon her finger. The three deformed sisters seated themselves round the room, like so many graven images, and all night not one of them opened her mouth. I'm not romancing, Hargrave; this is absolute fact. In the early morning a fearful thunder-storm broke out, one of the most violent I have ever known. The little garret burned blue with the lightning, and the thunder roared and rattled as if it were on the very roof of the house. It wasn't much of a lamp I had, and it was a queer thing when a spurt of lightning came to see those three twisted figures sitting round the walls, or to have the voice of my patient drowned by the booming of the thunder. By Jove, I don't mind telling you that there was a time when I nearly bolted from the room. All came right in the end, but I never heard the true story of the unfortunate beauty and her three crippled sisters.'

'That's the worst of these medical stories,' sighs the outsider. 'They never seem to have an end.'

'When a man is up to his neck in practice, my boy, he has no time to gratify his private curiosity. Things shoot across him and he gets a glimpse of them, only to recall them, perhaps, at some quiet moment like this. But I've always felt, Manson, that your line had as much of the terrible in it as any other.'

'More,' groans the alienist. 'A disease of the body is bad enough, but this seems to be a disease of the soul. Is it not a shocking thing – a thing to drive a reasoning man into absolute Materialism – to think that you may have a fine, noble fellow with every divine instinct and that some little vascular change, the dropping, we will say, of a minute spicule of bone from the inner table of his skull on to the surface of his brain may have the effect of changing him to a filthy and pitiable creature with every low and debasing tendency? What a satire an asylum is upon the majesty of man, and no less upon the ethereal nature of the soul.'

'Faith and hope,' murmurs the general practitioner.

'I have no faith, not much hope, and all the charity I can afford,' says the surgeon. 'When theology squares itself with the facts of life I'll read it up.'

'You were talking about cases,' says the outsider, jerking the ink down into his stylographic pen.

'Well, take a common complaint which kills many thousands every year, like G.P., for instance.'

'What's G.P.?'

'General practitioner,' suggests the surgeon with a grin.

'The British public will have to know what G.P. is,' says the alienist gravely. 'It's increasing by leaps and bounds, and it has the distinction of being absolutely incurable. General paralysis is its full title, and I tell you it promises to be a perfect scourge. Here's a fairly typical case now which I saw last Monday week. A young farmer, a splendid fellow, surprised his friends by taking a very rosy view of things at a time when the whole country-side was grumbling. He was going to give up wheat, give up arable land, too, if it didn't pay, plant two thousand acres of rhododendrons and get a monopoly of the supply for Covent Garden – there was no end to his schemes, all sane enough but just a bit inflated. I called at the farm, not to see him, but on an altogether different matter. Something about the man's way of talking struck me and I watched him narrowly. His lip had a trick of quivering, his words slurred themselves together, and so did his handwriting when he had occasion to draw up a small agreement. A closer inspection showed me that one of his pupils was ever so little larger than the other. As I left the house his wife came after me. "Isn't it splendid to see Job looking so well, doctor?" said she; "he's that full of energy he can hardly keep himself quiet." I did not say anything, for I had not the heart, but I knew that the fellow was as much condemned to death as though he were lying in the cell at Newgate. It was a characteristic case of incipient G.P.'

'Good heavens!' cries the outsider. 'My own lips tremble. I often slur my words. I believe I've got it myself.'

Three little chuckles come from the front of the fire.

'There's the danger of a little medical knowledge to the layman.'

'A great authority has said that every first year's student is suffering, in silent agony, from four diseases,' remarks the surgeon. 'One is heart disease, of course; another is cancer of the parotid. I forget the two other.'

'Where does the parotid come in?'

'Oh, it's the last wisdom tooth coming through!'

'And what would be the end of that young farmer?' asks the outsider.

'Paresis of all the muscles, ending in fits, coma and death. It may be a few months, it may be a year or two. He was a very strong young man and would take some killing.'

'By the way,' says the alienist, 'did I ever tell you about the first certificate I ever signed? I stood as near ruin then as a man could go.'

'What was it, then?'

'I was in practice at the time. One morning a Mrs Cooper called upon me and informed me that her husband had shown signs of delusions lately. They took the form of imagining that he had been in the army and had distinguished himself very much. As a matter of fact he was a lawyer and had never been out of England. Mrs Cooper was of opinion that if I were to call it might alarm him, so it was agreed between us that she should send him up in the evening on some pretext to my consulting-room, which would give me the opportunity of having a chat with him and, if I were convinced of his insanity, of signing his certificate. Another doctor had already signed, so that it only needed my concurrence to have him placed under treatment. Well, Mr Cooper arrived in the evening about half an hour before I had expected him, and consulted me as to some malarious symptoms from which he said that he suffered. According to his account he had just returned from the Abyssinian Campaign, and had been one of the first of the British forces to enter Magdala. No delusion could possibly be more marked, for he would talk of little else, so I filled in the papers without the slightest hesitation. When his wife arrived, after he had left, I put some questions to her to complete the form. "What is his age?" I asked. "Fifty," said she. "Fifty!" I cried. "Why, the man I examined could not have been more than thirty!" And so it came out that the real Mr Cooper had never called upon me at all, but that by one of those coincidences which take a man's breath away another Cooper, who really was a very distinguished young officer of artillery, had come in to consult me. My pen was wet to sign the paper when I discovered it,' says Dr Manson, mopping his forehead.

'We were talking about nerve just now,' observes the surgeon. 'Just after my qualifying I served in the Navy for a time, as I think you know. I was on the flag-ship on the West African Station, and I remember a singular example of nerve which came to my notice at that time. One of our small gunboats had gone up the Calabar river, and while there the surgeon died of coast fever. On the same day a man's leg was broken by a spar falling upon it, and it became quite obvious that it must be taken off above the knee if his life was to be saved. The young lieutenant who was in charge of the craft searched among the dead doctor's effects and laid his hands upon some chloroform, a hip-joint knife, and a volume of Grey's *Anatomy*. He had the man laid by the steward upon the cabin table, and with a picture of a cross section of the thigh in front of him he began to take off the limb. Every now and then, referring to the diagram, he would say: "Stand by with the lashings, steward. There's blood on the chart about here." Then he would jab with his knife until he cut the artery, and he and his assistant would tie it up before they went any further. In this way they gradually whittled the leg off, and upon my word they made a very excellent job of it. The man is hopping about the Portsmouth Hard at this day.

'It's no joke when the doctor of one of these isolated gunboats himself falls ill,' continues the surgeon after a pause. 'You might think it easy for him to prescribe for himself, but this fever knocks you down like a club, and you haven't strength left to brush a mosquito off your face. I had a touch of it at Lagos, and I know what I am telling you. But there was a chum of mine who really had a curious experience. The whole crew gave him up, and, as they had never had a funeral aboard the ship, they began rehearsing the forms so as to be ready. They thought that he was unconscious, but he swears he could hear every word that passed. "Corpse comin' up the 'atchway!" cried the cockney sergeant of Marines. "Present harms!" He was so amused, and so indignant, too, that he just made up his mind that he wouldn't be carried through that hatchway, and he wasn't, either.'

'There's no need for fiction in medicine,' remarks Foster, 'for the facts will always beat anything you can fancy. But it has seemed to me sometimes that a curious paper might be read at some of these meetings about the uses of medicine in popular fiction.'

'How?'

'Well, of what the folk die of, and what diseases are made most use of in novels. Some are worn to pieces, and others, which are equally common in real life, are never mentioned. Typhoid is fairly frequent, but scarlet fever is unknown. Heart disease is common, but then heart disease, as we know it, is usually the sequel of some foregoing disease, of which we never hear anything in the romance. Then there is the mysterious malady called brain fever, which always attacks the heroine after a crisis, but which is unknown under that name to the text-books. People when they are over-excited in novels fall down in a fit. In a fairly large experience I have never known anyone to do so in real life. The small complaints simply don't exist. Nobody ever gets shingles or quinsy, or mumps in a novel. All the diseases, too, belong to the upper part of the body. The novelist never strikes below the belt.'

'I'll tell you what, Foster,' says the alienist, 'there is a side of life which is too medical for the general public and too romantic for the professional journals, but which contains some of the richest human materials that a man could study. It's not a pleasant side, I am afraid, but if it is good enough for Providence to create, it is good enough for us to try and understand. It would deal with strange outbursts of savagery and vice in the lives of the best men, curious momentary weaknesses in the record of the sweetest women, known but to one or two, and inconceivable to the world around. It would deal, too, with the singular phenomena of waxing and of waning manhood, and would throw a light upon those actions which have cut short many an honoured career and sent a man to a prison when he should have been hurried to a consulting-room. Of all evils that may come upon the sons of men, God shield us principally from that one!'

'I had a case some little time ago which was out of the ordinary,' says the surgeon. 'There's a famous beauty in London Society – I mention no names – who used to be remarkable a few seasons ago for the very low dresses which she would wear. She had the whitest of skins, and most beautiful of shoulders, so it was no wonder. Then gradually the frilling at her neck lapped upwards and upwards, until last year she astonished every one by wearing quite a high collar at a time when it was completely out of fashion. Well, one day this very woman was shown into my consulting-room. When the footman was gone she suddenly tore off the upper part of her dress. "For God's sake do something for me!" she cried. Then I saw what the trouble was. A rodent ulcer was eating its way upwards, coiling on in its serpiginous fashion until the end of it was flush with her collar. The red streak of its trail was lost below the line of her bust. Year by year it had ascended and she had heightened her dress to hide it, until now it was about to invade her face. She had been too proud to confess her trouble, even to a medical man.'

'And did you stop it?'

'Well, with zinc chloride I did what I could. But it may break out again. She was one of those beautiful white-and-pink creatures who are rotten with struma. You may patch, but you can't mend.'

'Dear! dear! dear!' cries the general practitioner, with that kindly softening of the eyes which had endeared him to so many thousands. 'I suppose we mustn't think ourselves wiser than Providence, but there are times when one feels that something is wrong in the scheme of things. I've seen some sad things in my life. Did I ever tell you that case where Nature divorced a most loving couple? He was a fine young fellow, an athlete and a gentleman, but he overdid athletics. You know how the force that controls us gives us a little tweak to remind us when we get off the beaten track. It may be a pinch on the great toe if we drink too much and work too little. Or it may be a tug on our nerves if we dissipate energy too much. With the athlete, of course, it's the heart or the lungs. He had bad phthisis and was sent to Davos. Well, as luck would have it, she developed rheumatic fever, which left her heart very much affected. Now, do you see the dreadful dilemma in which those poor people found themselves? When he came below 4,000 feet or so, his symptoms became terrible. She could come up about 2,500, and then her heart reached its limit. They had several interviews half-way down the valley, which left them nearly dead, and at last, the doctors had to absolutely forbid it. And so for four years they lived within three miles of each other and never met. Every morning he would go to a place which over-looked the chalet in which she lived and would wave a great white cloth and she answer from below. They could see each other quite plainly with their field-glasses, and they might have been in different planets for all their chance of meeting.'

'And one at last died,' says the outsider.

'No, sir. I'm sorry not to be able to clinch the story, but the man recovered and is now a successful stockbroker in Drapers Gardens. The woman, too, is the mother of a considerable family. But what are you doing there?'

'Only taking a note or two of your talk.'

The three medical men laugh as they walk towards their overcoats.

'Why, we've done nothing but talk shop,' says the general practitioner. 'What possible interest can the public take in that?'

Rachel Naomi Remen

Rachel Naomi Remen – a cancer specialist and therapist – sees 'the practice of medicine as a spiritual path'. She is a pioneer of the holistic and more spiritual approach to healthcare, especially in life-threatening diseases such as cancer, and has counselled those with chronic and terminal illness for over 20 years. She herself has been a long-term sufferer from Crohn's disease. Her books on her clinical experiences, and her philosophy of life, include *Kitchen Table Wisdom: stories that heal* (1996) and *My Grandfather's Blessings: stories of strength, refuge and belonging* (2000). She is a clinical professor of family and community medicine at the University of California, San Francisco.

In his review of *Kitchen Table Wisdom*, Deepak Chopra wrote that the book shows how 'physicians can become healers by no longer remaining mere technicians of the human body, but by becoming alchemists of the soul'.

In the Gray Zone

by Rachel Naomi Remen

A woman with metastatic cancer once told me that through the experience of her illness she had discovered a basic truth. There are only two kinds of people in this world – those who are alive and those who are afraid. She had smiled at me and said that many of the people she had met who were afraid were doctors.

Perhaps such fear is a natural outcome of the wish to be in control. A patient whose physician told him several years ago that he had three months to live told me in bewilderment that the doctor had seemed 'satisfied' as he made this heart-stopping statement. 'He seemed sorry to be telling me this but he seemed pleased that he had the information to give me, almost as pleased as if he had told me that he had the right drug to eradicate my cancer. He told me of my death with an air of authority as if it were he who had decided when it would be and in doing so had somehow gained mastery over it. As if when he could not control my cancer, he could at least control the time of my death. I was angry for a long time, but I now think he was as out of control and vulnerable as I was. Too bad we could not have talked man to man on that level instead of reaching for a false certainty.'

Perhaps the most basic skill of the physician is the ability to have comfort with uncertainty, to recognize with humility the uncertainty inherent in all situations, to be open to the ever-present possibility of the surprising, the mysterious, and even the holy, and to meet people there.

The need for certainty is not just a problem for medical professionals. We wish for certainty as ardently as our doctors do, are seduced by it as profoundly and are as disappointed with the uncertain nature of the world. We all yearn for mastery. But mastery is always limited. Sooner or later we will come to the edge of all that we can control and find life, waiting there for us.

The wish to control floats like a buoy above the hidden reef of fear. More than any single thing, fear is the stumbling block to life's agenda. Perhaps it is only the things we fear that we wish to control. No one can serve life if they are unconsciously afraid of life. Life is process. When he was very old, Roberto Assagioli, the founder of psychosynthesis, reminded one of his young students of this: 'There is no certainty; there is only adventure,' he told this young man. 'Even stars explode.'

Part 2: Patients

In their eyes I am not a man, I am a patient.

Clive Sinclair

One has a greater sense of intellectual degradation after an interview with a doctor, than from any other human experience.

Alice James

Every patient, he said, provided two questions – firstly, what can be learnt from him and secondly what can be done for him.

Harvey Cushing

For disease will peer up over the hedge of health, with only its eyes showing.

John Stone

Renate Rubinstein

At the age of 47, the Dutch journalist Renate Rubinstein was diagnosed as having multiple sclerosis (MS). She had been working as a columnist on the Amsterdam weekly newspaper *Vrij Nederland*, writing under the pseudonym 'Tamar'. She was also the author of 20 books on various social and political topics. It took her ten years to come to terms with her disease sufficiently to write about it, and the resulting book *Take It and Leave It* – describing the inexorable advance of her illness, its impact on her life and her relationships, and her many interactions with doctors – became a major best-seller in Holland.

Rubinstein's book, with its wry speculations on life and death, is one of the most lucid ever written on physical disability and its encroaching effects on the individual. Throughout, its tone is clear-sighted and ironic, and without any trace of self-pity. As the disease waxes and wanes, disabling her body, but not her mind, she remarks on the paradox of MS, that 'when you are healthy you are not ill, but when you are ill you are healthy at the same time'.

Telling the Truth

by Renate Rubinstein

Should the doctor always give his patient the naked truth? That is, the name of the disease, the diagnosis?

The pros and cons of this question are many. The arguments have so often been repeated that they have lost their meaning for me. A patient wants to be able to trust his doctor, but at the same time he wants a truth which will reassure him. Other truths will cause resistance and resentment in the patient. Was that really necessary? What's the use? thinks the patient, who for that matter often does not believe the diagnosis just like that and begins by getting angry at the doctor before spreading his resentment to those around him and the world in general. Almost every sufferer of a chronic disease, mine or another, despises his first specialist, and I think this is because he was the bearer of bad news.

One thing I liked about my neurologist was that he had refused to tell me of his unfavourable findings. Maybe that was the basis for our friendly relationship later. He had chosen the easy way out, accepting the offer of a friend to act as an intermediary, but I did not find this cowardly. It was nice to know I meant so much to him he didn't dare tell me!

'It was difficult because you live alone,' he said later. 'But fortunately you have a sedentary profession. You are not an actress – if you were you would have to find a new occupation.' He is not the type to put on big compassionate humanitarian eyes. He is the type who always follows up an unpleasant truth with words of encouragement. A penny for the patient – that suited me fine. (What he really preferred talking about was exhibitions, concerts and new books, which I liked, although when I drove home I realized that once again I had learned nothing. Annie S., the writer, says that her doctors tend to tell her about their personal problems with wives or children. She is a motherly type, and her doctors love talking to her. Nevertheless, she says, she would prefer the information a patient expects from his doctor. Sometimes there is nothing much to say, I suggest with resignation. They don't know everything, they are waiting to see what happens. Annie wonders, she goes off to get me something from the kitchen – our doctors remain a mystery to us.)

In retrospect I think that, during my first visit – when my only fear was that he might think I was exaggerating – the neurologist already knew what I had probably got. There is a reflex action of the toes which the layman knows nothing about, but which is significant for the expert. Dressed in his white coat at the hospital (unlike the alternative doctor, the orthodox doctor doesn't wear a white coat in his office anymore), the neurologist practised the classical method on me: one examination after another, continuing uncertainty, and waiting for yet another test that might give a definite answer. Even a month after I left the hospital, he continued with this method. He still wasn't certain. For a definite diagnosis I would have to return to hospital to be x-rayed with contrasting fluids in my spinal marrow. I never went again; ninety percent certainty (or was it eighty?) was sufficient for me.

The method that is practised with all diseases, and cancer in particular, has been called 'the system of hope'. I find there is much to be said for this method, but people who believe in human dignity and the benefits of sincerity object to it, and there is something to be said for that as well, I think. The objections come mainly from psychoanalysts, who would prefer to help hospital patients in their own way. Here they encounter the scepticism of medical specialists whose approach has been tested by experience. And even if it is true that their method suits them better, they feel that it is better for the patient as well. They don't see much benefit in psychological treatment. 'Medical treatment itself, as exorcism, is medical psychological treatment,' writes Abram de Swaan in his book on the Welfare State.

Let me quote one passage from this book:

'From the start, the treatment offers the patients a way of living with their disease and their fears. Something can be done about the frightening inexorable process – there are experts, treatments, cancer institutes. The treatment also offers a time perspective of its own: instead of the threatening feeling of a fate that will unfold over an indefinite period of time, a structured and fixed timetable of referrals and interventions is established.

'The patient is not waiting for the terrible end, but is awaiting the outcome of an operation in two weeks. Instead of his frightening fate, successive favourable and unfavourable reports on the effects of different therapies absorb the attention: the treatment breaks the vision of doom down to a series of good and bad results, all in an orderly and measured time perspective. With this treatment schedule, thoughts of death are postponed time and again.'

I cite this disillusioning passage without qualms, because I know from my own experience that patients are not easily disillusioned. The unconscious, the existence of which is so often contested, is there. I have experienced it myself. Like a heavenly mother it protects you against hard blows; even the rudest modern purveyors of total truth can't break through it. When my neurologist began a long-winded description of my disease, my thoughts strayed at once. Have it your way, I thought, I know it's the sleeping pills. It's my own fault. I will stop taking Mogadon and will spend three weeks lying in bed without sleep. In short, this verbiage didn't interest me. I did not listen. My unconscious self protected me. Illusions cannot be taken away by 'them', at least not immediately, and not for good, they belong to the psychic nature of the beast to whom truth is of no concern.

There is yet another aspect to this revealing of truth. People find it damned annoying if others know something about them that they don't even know themselves. The first thing I did after hearing 'the truth', was to call Jaap Q., who was then my G.P. He had come to visit me in hospital and had sat silently and gloomily beside my bed. 'So you knew all along what was wrong with me,' I cried indignantly. 'I still don't know what you've got,' said Jaap. The nurses, the physiotherapist, whom I saw daily, also knew nothing. They had not deceived me when they said they did not know, and they had not been pitying me over their coffee cups. I was not the only one in whom the neurologist had not confided. I found that a relief. There was plenty of injury, but insult had not been added. How tactful of the medical profession.

Ruth Picardie

Ruth Nadine Picardie was 32 years old when she was diagnosed as having breast cancer. She had been married for only two years, and had one-year-old twins, Joe and Lola. She was born in 1964 in Reading, the daughter of South African émigrés to Britain, and her middle name was after the South African novelist Nadine Gordimer. She studied social anthropology at Cambridge University, and then worked as a journalist on the *Guardian* and *Independent* newspapers, and also as a freelance writer for a range of periodicals – from *Vogue* to the *Sunday Telegraph* magazine. After her cancer was diagnosed in 1996, she underwent extensive treatment, but despite this, the condition advanced inexorably. It soon became clear that her condition was terminal. In her last year, Ruth wrote five columns on her illness for the *Life* magazine section of the *Observer* newspaper, and also had an extensive e-mail correspondence with friends and well-wishers from all over the world. After her death in 1998, these columns and e-mails were collected into a book, *Before I Say Goodbye*, by her husband, Matt Seaton, and her sister, Justine Picardie.

Observer Life, 3 August 1997

by Ruth Picardie

It's official, then. After nine months of talking bravely about 50:50 survival rates . . . of bone disease being a really 'good' form of secondary breast cancer . . . of a new, 'natural' chemotherapy regime which is showing really promising results . . . of confident declarations of recovery from my healer and Chinese doctor . . . I now have a brain tumour. Oh, and, by the way, the lurgy is advancing rapidly into my liver and lungs, so there's no point in continuing with treatment. So no more false dawns, no more miracle cures, no more *Alien*-style eruptions of disease (I now have a 'full house' of secondary breast cancer sites – or 'mets', as we professionals like to say). The bottom line is, I'm dying.

Frankly, the brain tumour didn't come as a huge surprise. I've been getting sicky headaches, lasting three or four days, and wiggly lights appearing at the periphery of my vision. Plus, I didn't really believe the doctors back in May, when they noticed a weird lesion on my brain which, they assured me, had nothing to do with the breast cancer. Yeah, right, I've got a rare neurological condition, too.

Still, I'm pretty scared. Not that breast cancer has been a picnic so far: all those hats I made people buy when I thought I was going bald and then felt guilty about not wearing; the fear of getting a new, different cancer from radiotherapy to the breast (as if!); losing the will to wash the kitchen floor. Hey, you've heard it all before. But having a brain tumour is not fun.

My oncologist tells me not to worry, that the right front lobe is pretty useless, as far as bits of the brain go. Which is reassuring. Then I read my book – snappily titled *Breast Cancer* – and it says, 'Secondary tumours in the brain which produce a rise in pressure within the skull can lead to headaches or to specific neurological signs, such as disorders of speech or movement and epileptic fits. These may also arise from damage by the tumour itself, which can also cause various disorders of mental or nervous system functions, including epilepsy and dementia.' Great. I'm going to die, but I'm going to go bonkers first.

Actually, my oncologist tells me that the liver disease is going to get me before the brain tumour, which is reassuring. 'Secondaries in the liver can cause nausea,' explains my book, 'loss of appetite and weight loss as well as the intense itching and yellow coloration of the skin typical of jaundice . . . Liver tumours which expand rapidly can produce severe pain.' Turning into a bruised lemon is, I reckon, better than going mad.

But whichever bit of my failing anatomy collapses first, I'm pretty upset. What hurts most is losing the future. I won't be there to clap when my beloved babies learn to write their names; I won't see them learn to swim, or go to school, or play the piano; I won't be able to read them *Pippi Longstocking*, or kiss their innocent knees when they fall off their bikes. (All right, so I won't have to clean pooh out of the bath, or watch *Pingu* for the 207th time, or hose spinach sauce off the floor.) Then there's the really important stuff: I won't be able to watch the fourth series of *ER* (will Ross and Hathaway live happily ever after?); I'll never know if the pregnancy stretchmarks on my legs would have disappeared without surgery; I haven't got time to grow my patchy, chemotherapy crop into a halo of life-before-cancer curls.

Plus, there's all the stuff I've got to do now: the agonising task of compiling 'memory boxes' for Lola and Joe (how do you write the definitive love letter to a partly imaginary child?); cleaning out the bathroom cabinet; getting into a size 12.

Meanwhile, it's bloody tough living in limbo, not knowing exactly how long I've got left. Do I get a four-month or a 12-month prescription prepayment certificate? Do I bother stocking up on Sisley day facial scrub, when I've got a whole tube of La Prairie night cleanser left? Can I justify going to the next Ghost sale, and who gets my black skirt after my death?

Still, I'm trying to look on the bright side. Missing the Greenwich Millennium exhibition is not a major source of grief. Matt gets to keep all the guilt if – when push comes to oratory – Lola and Joe end up going to private school (the New Labour Academy of Hypocrisy). And it's one way of solving the post-feminist, double-barrelled, what-surname-to-give-the-kids dilemma. (His. Who wants to be named after a dead post-feminist?)

And, looking back, I don't have many regrets. I was privileged to live through the era of John Frieda restructuring serum, which revolutionised life for women with curly hair. I loved my Matt. We loved our Lola and Joe.

And the future will get on just fine without me. OK, so Matt never waters the garden, which means the wisteria is hardly likely to make the next century. Plus, he never gets up in the night to put blankets back on the kids, but nobody ever died of cold in a centrally heated house. Otherwise, I think life will continue just fine. It's just that I'll miss it so.

Rachel Clark

I had no idea what cancer involved until I was suddenly thrown in to the middle of the cancer world,

wrote Rachel Clark, at the end of her book – written for the benefit of other cancer victims, and for the doctors that treated them.

She was born in London in 1970, one of twins, and was educated at the University of Bristol, where she studied psychology, later training as an occupational psychologist. At the age of 25, while working in Australia for a two-year period as a management consultant, Rachel developed a series of vague symptoms, and was then diagnosed as having a rare cancer of her nasal sinuses – a rhabdomyosarcoma. By the time it was diagnosed, the cancer had already spread. She underwent three years of treatment – initially in Sydney, and then eventually back in London. It was after her return to the UK in 1996 that she began to write a detailed account of her experiences of the disease, and of her medical treatments. After her death in 1998, her account was published as a book, *A Long Walk Home* (2002), which includes an Epilogue by her twin sister, Naomi Jefferies.

The extract that follows is the first chapter of her book. It tells of her earliest symptoms, and then of her shock at hearing her true diagnosis and its likely prognosis.

Inside Out and Upside Down: diagnosis

by Rachel Clark

I could feel it everywhere. I inhaled its smell, let its tastes run across my tongue, its sounds echo in my ears. I could sense its warmth spreading across the city, a smooth and golden treacle flowing through the streets, over buildings and houses, and onwards into the sea. A brilliant sun scorched the jacaranda trees which showered the city with a confetti of gentle purple flowers. Blue skies reflected in the harbour's mirror as it sparkled and glistened like liquid diamonds. The eye could skim across its gleaming surface and climbing, continue up and up to the pinnacle of the skyline. The skyscrapers shone, radiating beads of a harder light, scattering beams in random directions as the piercing rays reflected off the thousands of symmetrical windowpanes. Rows and columns of the city's transparent mask. The mask of Sydney, as it welcomed the summer.

I too, as the city, was melting into summer. Indulgently I sucked in its heat through every pore. With growing anticipation I awaited its promises of mornings at the beach merging into balmy days and evenings at streetside cafés. Sunny days, days full of friends and fun, games of tennis, swimming in the sea. Days to fill with my own idealistic hopes, dreams and plans. My life was good and deep down I knew it. I lived in a characteristic terraced house in the city's leafy eastern suburbs, sharing with two wonderful girlfriends and a big red cat. We had a warm and welcoming home that was, more often than not, full of friends and laughter. I had a good job with an international company and, at my own request, I had been granted my dream secondment from London – two years in Australia. I had made a colourful group of interesting and enjoyable friends, I had the time to do the sport and exercise I loved, my life was full of new adventures and opportunities. Everything seemed rosy to me. Nothing in my experiences could have led me to imagine, even in my wildest dreams, the challenges that lay ahead of me. Could anything have prepared me for the biggest, highest, widest hurdle of my life? I was 25 years old. I was diagnosed with cancer.

Hindsight reminds me that there were some 'warning symptoms', but hindsight is, of course, a wonderful thing. Nothing I was experiencing appeared to me to be particularly out of the ordinary. I'd been pretty tired for a while but I had all the explanations. I had just moved house, there had been a few hiccups in my personal life, and, of course, there was that constant sinusitis that was proving so difficult to shift. It must, I reasoned, be the combination of several minor events that were getting on top of me. I had paid a number of visits to a GP culminating in a vast array of antibiotics and nasal sprays. I was on great terms with the local pharmacist, probably stocking a greater range of medications in my medicine cabinet than he did on his tower of shelves. My GP was beginning to despair of me.

'Maybe you're allergic to Sydney,' he suggested unhelpfully, 'maybe you should consider moving.' Regarding this advice as impractical, I tried a different GP. He again tried a further range of pills and sprays to no avail. 'One of my friends with awful sinuses tried squirting garlic oil up his nose,' he tried in desperation, 'you could always try that.'

He began an elaborate description of how his friend had constructed his personal garlic spray, but, sensing my rather lukewarm response, trailed off, deciding not to pursue his line of discussion any further. I did not know what to try. My own rather simplistic 'leave it and it'll go away' approach appeared to have as little validity as my GP's garlic oil. I had to find something. Life was becoming a struggle. Everything was such hard work. I wasn't strolling through every day in the sun, but jogging, uphill with a full pack, in the rain.

Being visibly below par led my secretary to suggest that I visit her acupuncturist. I decided to try; after all it sounded more feasible than the garlic. The dainty Chinese doctor had a shrunken, wrinkled face, its lines hinting at a lifetime of hidden stories. He was small and silent, he even moved around noiselessly as if he floated above the floor's surface, a soundless hovercraft. My secretary had assured me that he had worked miracles for her. I sat in the waiting room with nervous interest until he ushered me through to a small cubicle containing a doctor's couch covered with a crisp white sheet. He motioned to me to lie down and then, very gently, he placed delicate needles in my hands and face. Tinkly Chinese music echoed in my ears as I peacefully drifted off, sleeping my way through an afternoon that should have been spent industriously at work. I had enjoyed the rest but, overall, I still wasn't any better. Maybe I needed a holiday, just to get away from the pressures of everyday life? I could test out the GP's 'allergy to Sydney' theory and my own suspicion that maybe work stresses were getting to me and that I just needed a break. I successfully discredited both by a sailing trip in the Whitsunday Islands. The day after I returned I was back in my GP's surgery.

'I think I should see a specialist' I blurted out.

I quite surprised myself. I didn't really know what sort of 'specialist' existed, let alone what they would actually be able to do for me. I wondered if I was really making a bit too much fuss over the whole thing.

Two weeks later I was sitting in a chair in a Macquarie Street (Sydney's version of Harley Street) consulting room. It was a fairly small room, well filled by dark, old style wooden furniture. The ear, nose and throat specialist had peered up my nose through a circular hole in a metal disk attached to a band around his head. What a strange looking instrument, I thought. Seeing little of any note he had anaesthetised my nose with a disgusting tasting anaesthetic spray and then inserted an endoscope (telescopic probe) up my nose. I wriggled in discomfort.

'Hmm' he pondered, 'I can't see much but I had difficulty getting the endoscope through into your sinuses. I think you should have a scan.'

I felt a bit of a sham really. Surely I didn't need to waste people's time by having what I regarded as serious medical attention. I had never had a 'proper' scan before. Dr Haxell seemed a nice man who, we had discovered while I was describing my work to him, was the father of a friend and colleague. I didn't want to bother him with my minor medical concerns. I was sure that he had more important things to deal with.

Fast forward one week. I was back again, in that cluttered consulting room, clutching a large manila folder full of darkly coloured scans. I sat on the edge of my chair trying not to seem impatient, as Dr Haxell carefully studied the scans.

'Well, you're certainly not being neurotic' he said.

I was relieved. At least I wasn't wasting his time being a hypochondriac. He started pointing to the scans, highlighting a light coloured patch that appeared to be an obstruction in the sinus cavities on the right hand side of my face. I learned that sinuses were not just sinuses and that my major blockage was in what was called my ethmoid sinus.

'What is it?' I asked shakily.

'Well, it is probably just a mucocoele or polyps' he said 'although the image looks like it could be a solid mass. It's hard to tell.'

The significance of the latter half of the statement was lost on me as I contemplated the words mucocoele and polyps. Presumably I should know what they meant, I searched my head for definitions but resorted to nodding my head in agreement.

'We'll have to operate.'

His words stopped my searching. Operate. I'd never had an operation in my life. I couldn't think of many friends who'd had operations either. I'd had my teeth taken out under gas when I was nine years old and I'd found that distressing enough. I was surprisingly shaken. I wandered back through the morning sunshine in the general direction of work, immersed so deeply in my own thoughts I could have drowned in them. An operation. I didn't know what to think. I crossed the street in a daze. Not usually a teary person, I was on the verge of crying. I sat in the park trying to pull myself together. I was irritated by my weakness. 'It's just a small operation' I told myself. 'Don't be so pathetic, you can deal with this.' I sat in the sun until the heat of its rays relaxed me and I felt a little more composed before I headed back to work, scans snug in their manila folder underneath my arm.

I had never had many dealings with the medical profession or the medical system before. I had no idea what would or should happen next. Dr Haxell only operated privately but recommended that a colleague of his, Dr Stanton, perform my relatively minor operation. I waited to be given a date. Expecting, through my work in the business world, a fairly rapid response, I was dismayed to discover that Dr Stanton would be unable to operate for another 6–8 weeks. For reasons I don't fully understand, I was convinced that I couldn't wait that long. I was rapidly feeling worse but felt unable to justify so much sick leave. How could I take two months off work to wait for an operation to correct a minor sinus problem? After a tearful phone call to my sister she persuaded me to ring Dr Stanton and explain to him why I felt such an urgent need for attention. Eventually I tracked him down and blurted out my situation. He was, he explained, very busy with conferences, scheduled operations and such like. They were, he pointed out, trying to help me but I would just have to wait. I was obviously irritating him. Something inside me wouldn't accept 'you'll have to wait' for an answer. 'What if I see you privately?' I persisted. He agreed that I could do that and asked me to bring my scans to him between operations at his hospital that week.

So I set off again, manila folder in hand. Dr Stanton found me as a somewhat lost young woman wandering around by the lifts, identifying me by the non-hospital folder of scans. He had, I expect, hoped to allay my fears and concerns for immediate treatment by a quick five minute consultation. A serious faced and mild mannered man, he studied my scans with intense concentration.

'I think you were right to come in, I'll operate on Monday.'

Today was Friday. I would only need to be in hospital overnight, he assured me, it was a minor procedure. 'At least it will all be over soon' I comforted myself internally. Then I would begin to feel better again.

I didn't really have enough time to panic. The weekend was suddenly over. My brother had arrived from England for a year of 'doing Oz' having just graduated from university and in no great hurry to get himself locked into a career and a nine to five routine. Our reunion after a year was only slightly marred by my minor hospital stay looming over the edge of the weekend. For his part, Nick was pleased that he'd get my bed for a day or two rather than the rather battered sofa which was the available alternative, as well as sole use of my car. We drank beer and ate sushi, much to his disgust (the sushi not the beer). It was a welcome distraction to have him around.

Hospital admissions seem to be a slow and complicated process. Within a few hours I'd had a taste of how alienating hospital procedures could be. I sat in my allocated ward feeling very much in everybody's way. The two old ladies in the ward appeared to be part of the furniture. I sat watching them, imagining that I had been transported, an invisible intruder, into a scene from a rather bizarre comedy. Eventually, a disinterested nurse came to ask me some admission questions, then someone else asked me the same things all over again. I'd already begun counting the hours until I could go home. I began to feel quite miserable, until the anaesthetist appeared and life suddenly became more bearable. Dr McCullen, I still remember his name although I only saw him this once, wore bright red socks and a big smile. He was friendly and open, answering lots of my questions and explaining carefully what he was going to do. His questioning over, he disappeared, reappearing again in the operating theatre where he jokingly explained his reasons for being an anaesthetist until I went under. The last thing I remember was laughing with him and one of the surgical nurses. It helped to blunt the edge of my fear.

The first person I remember on coming round was someone by the name of Heather with a pink hat and a white clinical coat. I don't know who she was but she soon faded out of my consciousness, to be replaced, some hours later, by the surgeon's registrar, Dr Reynolds. I was still pretty groggy and my mouth was sore and stiff. She began to ask how I was feeling. Even before I interrupted her with the expected 'So what did you find?' I knew it was not a mucocoele or polyps, whatever they actually were. Usually optimistic and positive I had a gut feeling that something wasn't right.

'It was a solid mass' she told me.

They had done a biopsy and, when they had the results, they'd be able to let me know what it was. My mouth was sore, she explained, because they'd had to drill through my top jaw, above my right hand incisors, to remove a bung of glue-like mucus. The mass was blocking the connecting passages between the sinuses. I was in no frame of mind to ask questions. I just nodded vaguely and drifted back into a less than comfortable oblivion.

My fit and healthy body stood me in good stead. It had only been a minor procedure and within a week I was up and about and feeling rapidly better. The pressure from my sinuses was noticeably less and I began to believe that, whatever my problem was, 'they', the medical profession, were well on the way to sorting it all out for me. The next step would be the pathology results and then, well, the worst could surely be another minor operation restoring me to my rightful state of, in the belief of most people my age, everlasting health and immortality.

My knowledge of Sydney was still not particularly extensive. I'd been there for a year but really had little concept of a large proportion of the sprawling city. I'd unintentionally restricted my movements to the areas where I worked, lived and visited the still novel beaches. Hopefully requesting directions to Dr Stanton's consulting rooms prompted Sarah, one of my dearest and kindest friends, to offer to accompany me. She was convinced, with some experience of my navigating skills as justification, that I would get horribly lost. She also thought I could do with the company. Independently minded, I would happily have gone alone but learned that day of the value of having support and an extra pair of ears on hand. We still did, duly, get slightly lost but arrived at Dr Stanton's consulting room right on time. Dr Stanton seemed rather rushed and distracted. Maybe his clinic was very full that morning? I was surprised by his manner compared to the kind and helpful man I had met in the hospital. He was reluctant to make eye contact, his manner was strangely awkward and he was hesitant as to where to begin.

'Are the pathology results back?' I asked.

'The preliminary tests have been run and their findings necessitated further tests, I'm afraid.'

'What are they testing for?' Sarah and I asked in unison.

He talked a little more vaguely about the possibilities. I think that he did use the word tumour in this discussion but tumour, to me, meant little more than mucocoele or polyps had meant a few weeks earlier. I was rapidly feeling the need for a medical dictionary or five years at medical school. I asked if he had any idea what the pathology might show.

'One of five things' he replied cryptically, 'three of which we could do something about. Do you have any questions?'

'Yes. Yes' I screamed inside my head. 'I have hundreds of questions. What have I got? What is wrong with me?' Nothing came out.

'When will the pathology results be available?' asked Sarah, taking control of the conversation that I had relinquished. Next week, he thought, but he would be away at a conference. He suggested that we contact Dr Reynolds, his registrar, who would be able to give us the results. My mind was blank as we were hastily ushered out of the room. We'd been in there for less than ten minutes. I was still none the wiser. What was wrong with me? What did I have?

We sat in the car, side by side.

'Sarah, what exactly is a tumour?' my frozen mind began to thaw. 'I mean tumours, they can be all sorts of things can't they, malignant and benign.' She nodded in agreement.

'He'd have said if it was malignant' she comforted.

'But he wouldn't look at us properly' I worried, 'he was so uncomfortable with us.'

'Maybe he just hasn't got good people skills' she countered.

So round and round we went trying to understand the snippets of information that we had been fed. I cried and once I was crying I couldn't stop. Tears of fear mixed with tears of confusion and anxiety, going over again and again the things that Dr Stanton had said, the things that he hadn't said and the way he had acted. I was so grateful that Sarah was able to drive home. I would have been totally incapable of navigating myself to the bottom of my own garden path. The drive home seemed to have grown by miles and miles in the hour since we had made the outward journey.

Dr Reynolds was a young woman, only a few years older than I was. She'd had a pleasant, professional and slightly detached manner during our previous encounter at the hospital. I had rather liked her. As I and my flatmate Emily walked down the hospital corridor to see her we were laughing to ourselves. Two young women laughing about a now long forgotten joke. We were surprised to see Dr Reynolds waiting to greet us, I was already getting used to spending a significant proportion of my time in waiting rooms. She ushered us through to a cluttered consulting room, with too many chairs and a plethora of rather dubious looking medical implements. I recognised some of the ENT instruments from Dr Haxell's rooms. We all sat down and chatted, exchanging social pleasantries for a while.

'So, what did the path. results show? Do you know what it is?' I asked, trying to get down to the issue that had been gnawing at my mind constantly for over a week.

'I don't think it will mean that much to you' she replied.

She sat stiffly in her chair and was obviously ill at ease.

'Now' she continued, 'obviously the first question you will have is how long have you got' she looked directly at me 'and I'm afraid I can't tell you.'

I was confused. What was she talking about? I looked at my friend, her expression was one of equal confusion.

'I'm sorry' I started haltingly, 'I don't understand what you mean. Do you mean how long is it going to take until I'm better? How long the treatment is going to take.'

'No' she hesitated, 'I meant how long have you got to live' she paused 'and I'm afraid I can't tell you that because I'm not an oncologist.'

Here was another medical word I was expected to understand. What was an 'oncologist', and why wasn't one here, whatever they were? I felt more acutely than ever the need for that medical dictionary. A few moments turned into an eternity before she spoke again. 'I have seen these tumours before in children, but never in an adult.' Half-formed questions tumbled around inside my head like washing in a drier, wafting around but never able to get out. I looked up and saw that she was as shaken as I was. How difficult it must be to tell someone who, for all intents and purposes could easily be you, that they have cancer and that you think they are going to die. Hesitantly, I opened the door to the drier in my head. To each poorly articulated question that stumbled out of my mouth she seemed to answer 'I don't know, I'm not an oncologist'; she was right, she wasn't, where was this elusive beast? I asked her to write down the pathology results so that I could telephone Dr Haxell. Maybe he would be able to help me.

'Come back on Monday morning' she told me.

Her parting remark stuck in my mind.

'Please don't go and jump off the Harbour Bridge.'

At least she didn't attempt to tell me to 'have a nice weekend'.

'As much bloody use as a cardboard cut out' Emily muttered as we sat in a traffic jam.

'She didn't know that I didn't know I had cancer' I repeated. 'She didn't know.'

Had I misunderstood Dr Stanton? Had he told me? If he had, both Sarah and I had missed it. He'd mentioned tumour, so this was a serious tumour, malignant. It was cancer. I sat in the Friday night traffic, tears rolling down my face without really noticing. No one was giving me answers. I felt numb. I wished someone would just give me the complete picture. All I knew was that I had some unpronounceable cancer. I wanted information. What did it mean? What was going to happen to me? Was there any treatment? Was I going to die? Someone must know. The tumble drier of my mind had been overloaded. The thoughts were all getting tangled up with each other. It was in danger of blowing up.

We reached home, my safe home, with a newly festive Christmas wreath on the door. It made a stark contrast to the shock and utter helplessness, I had to find out what this all really meant. I sat down and tried to compose myself, to think rationally. I needed information. Could Dr Haxell help me? I hesitated to bother him at the weekend but . . . there was nobody else, I was desperate, I had to know what was going on. Forcing myself to stay calm and breathe slowly, I picked up the receiver and dialled.

'I've got something I can't even say' I blurted out as soon as he answered. 'I don't know what it is and they can't seem to tell me.'

I mispronounced my way through the pathology findings while he listened patiently at the other end. He was very calm and kind.

'Why don't you come round for a drink with us' he offered 'and we'll talk about it.'

My flatmates drove me over, they also wanted to know. He welcomed us in and sat us down around the dining room table with a bottle of wine. He proceeded to give us a technical, medical, but clear explanation of my disease. An alveolar rhabdomyosarcoma in my ethmoid sinus (it took me at least two weeks to learn how to say it). He gave us a lot of time to ask questions, however basic they seemed and, most importantly, he gave me hope that a cure was possible. 'Frequent mitosis', he pointed out, meant that although the tumour was growing quickly it would also respond to treatments quickly as they acted on dividing cells. He did not send me off, as the hospital had, to a weekend of extreme anxiety and panic, but gave me sleeping tablets, support and a hug. He responded to my needs as a human being, not as a problematic patient who could be put on hold over the weekend.

That night I called some friends who came straight over. We laughed and talked until the small hours. I washed my sleeping tablets down with champagne. I felt safer with people around me, their normality seemed to cushion me from the very abnormal and unreal situation in which I found myself. I imagined myself drowning in a champagne glass, smothered by the bubbles. I could hardly believe what had happened. Everything felt more and more unreal as I floundered through the weekend. I tried so hard to tell my mother and father calmly and rationally. I felt it was my 'duty' to tell them but I didn't have the information to answer their questions. I didn't want to panic and upset them or want them to be on the next plane out to Australia. I didn't really know what I wanted because I didn't know what I was dealing with. I spoke to my aunt and to my godfather, hoping that they could give my parents some support. I could not deal with my parents' fear as well as my own.

Some people gave me hope, including a family friend in England who was an oncologist. He had little experience of my particular form of cancer, and he hadn't seen my scans, but he thought that my chances should be quite good. 'High cure rates' he had thought. Others buried me deeper in the pit of despair, their own worries piling in mounds on my shoulders, on top of my own. Some had stories of miraculous cures. My sights were focused on Monday, I was marking off time until I could go back to the hospital. Surely then someone would give me some answers.

As I felt myself sinking, support rose up and cradled me from all directions, supporting me as dolphins support their injured companions. Sarah's mother, Geraldine, a highly experienced nurse, drove down to Sydney to come to the hospital with me. A wonderfully warm and sensible person, she was able to offer me practical help and advice. She came round to collect me early because, as she told me, 'I want to tell you some of the things they may tell you in the hospital before we get there, so that I can explain them and they don't shock you.' She talked to me about chemotherapy, about radiotherapy and about removing the tumour surgically. She also outlined some of the side effects. Chemotherapy, should I have it, could make me infertile. I had never questioned my fertility. I had always assumed that when I wanted children I would be able to have them. Then again I had taken many things for granted, including my life. In my work as a 'change management consultant' I had helped businesses assimilate organisational changes. In our own form of jargon we described the condition resulting from an excess of changes as experiencing 'change overload'. At this point people became totally saturated and could not assimilate any more change. I could have applied the label to myself and it would have fitted like a glove. Too many new and strange things were happening to me. How could my life have altered so rapidly? I felt confused and scared, I wasn't really able to process what had happened so far, yet there was so much more to come. How was I going to take it all in?

Dr Stanton was waiting for us at the hospital. Once again he made very little contact with any of us. He was very awkward and uncomfortable, nervously pacing around the room, not sitting. He began to talk us through the scans, glad to have something to focus on other than our faces. He was busily losing himself, and us, in his technical explanations when the door opened and he was interrupted by the arrival of two younger looking men. They were introduced to us as oncologists, so there was one mystery solved for me at least. They spoke together, briefly and inaudibly, my straining ears could pick up nothing.

Dr Stanton asked us to leave so that they could discuss my case in more detail. What were they going to say that they didn't want us to hear? We stood in a confused huddle in the corridor, waiting for someone to take control of the situation, a small herd of sheep waiting for a sheep dog. We began walking, desperate for something to do, wandering aimlessly up and down the hospital corridor, the rhythm of our steps counting out the minutes. Eventually, the door reopened and we were hastily ushered back in and seated in a line. Dr Stanton could not have exited more quickly if someone had shouted fire. I felt that in his eyes I was already dead. Maybe he should have taken the measurements for my coffin before he left, to save time later. The radiotherapist followed a close second. We were left with the medical oncologist, Dr Norton. The atmosphere felt much calmer. He sat down and made eye contact with us all. He told us up front that we had as much time as we needed. At last, I thought, someone to answer my questions. He explained that the scans showed a reasonably large tumour in my ethmoid sinus but that they wouldn't be sure of the extent of the disease until they had carried out a range of further tests. Some of the tests that he mentioned I had come across. Others were further foreign medical jargon. They needed bone scans, an MRI scan, a bone marrow biopsy, blood tests, a lumbar puncture to test my spinal fluid and a biopsy of the lump in my neck that I had assumed was a resurgence of my glandular fever. It had not occurred to me that the disease could have spread. I attempted to digest this news. He moved on, explaining the treatment. I would definitely need chemotherapy and, later on, some ray treatment. It was impossible to be specific, he told us, until they had the results of further tests. It was all very well talking about treatment options and further tests but there was one burning question that I had to bring myself to ask.

'You can cure this, can't you?' I looked straight at him.

'Well' he paused, 'we can have a go.'

I needed more than this.

'How likely is it that you can cure this?'

He hesitated, not wanting to go down this avenue of discussion.

'It's hard to put a figure on it, but' he paused 'on a scale of 1–100 it's at the lower end of the scale.'

This conversation seemed unreal to me, as if I was a fly on the wall listening in.

'How low?' I ventured.

'10–25%, depending on the outcome of the tests.'

Sarah squeezed my hand, Geraldine and Emily closed in around me. I don't remember much more about the consultation, just numbness, but when we left I found it difficult to walk. The car seemed to be a long way away.

Someone had just told me that I was probably going to die, and die soon. I looked down at my smooth tanned skin, at the flesh on my arms; these were healthy limbs, this was a healthy body. Other than a tumour my body was fit and well. How could my 'healthy' body just die? What would happen if I died? The world would go on much the same as before but without me. I felt so alive, so here, how could I not exist? It would be, I thought, rather like moving from London to Sydney. The lives of my friends and family in England, of which I had been a part, still went on, but without me. They would all still be here, breathing, walking around, getting on with their lives and I, well I would be somewhere else. I couldn't quite imagine it.

I tried not to be left alone with my thoughts. I was woefully ill-equipped to deal with them. I was in total shock yet trying to deal with questions about my mortality. I took comfort in the people who emerged to support me, my brother, my twin sister, Naomi, who flew up from Adelaide where she was living, the friends around me. Unfortunately, there is only room for one in an MRI machine. Before I was admitted to hospital an outpatient MRI scan (Magnetic Resonance Imaging) was arranged for me. I was accompanied by my wonderful Scottish friend Ralph. Alone with my thoughts for the first time in a claustrophobic tunnel with a great imitation of an earthquake going on around my head was too much for me. I wriggled out of the tunnel and burst into tears.

'What you need is a holiday' the technician advised me. 'I had a holiday last month, went to Bali, made me feel much better about all my problems' which she went on to tell me about in great detail.

'I can't go on holiday, I've got cancer' I told her once she'd finished her chronicle of woes.

'Oh' she said, and disappeared out of the room to summon Ralph.

I would have loved a holiday, a holiday away from the nightmare I had found myself in, but it didn't seem to be high up on my list of possible options. A second attempt at the scan, with headphones and Ralph holding my hand up the tunnel (until the blood supply was totally cut off he tells me, prompting various Billy Connolly jokes) proved more palatable and the scan was completed.

This was to be the beginning of the long line of explorations that my body was required to submit to. Admission to hospital took me away from the familiar and into a totally alien environment. I was no longer the Rachel in my own definition of self, I wasn't the strong and independent person I had thought myself to be, I was Rachel Clark, cancer patient, the girl with the rhabdomyosarcoma. I hated the hospital tags that I felt institutionalised me and robbed me of my individuality. I had a whirl of appointments that I defy any socialite to better. I met the social worker, the nursing team, what felt like an entire rugby side of different registrars and various other medico-types who appeared in my room at random. To each and every person I asked the same question. 'What can I do to help myself get well? What do other people do that works?' I desperately wanted to grasp hold of the situation, to win back some of the control that had been taken away from me. Now I knew what was wrong with me I wanted to be able to fix it. My need for control and understanding increased as my sense of alienation and confusion grew. Every test they wanted to do on me hurt, and each was new and upsetting. The lumbar puncture, taking a sample of my spinal fluid to determine whether the tumour had gone through into the brain, required me to lie flat on my back for 24 hours. That was quickly followed by a bone marrow biopsy in my hip. I knew that this would hurt, it is not possible to anaesthetise bone. I was scared.

'Do lie still. You're making it difficult for me' complained the registrar who was performing the procedure.

'Sorry' I apologised. Difficult for him, how difficult did he think it was for me?

Although I did feel pain I was sedated and, in reality, it was probably more painful for my sister and brother, Naomi and Nick, to watch my fear and discomfort, that is until, they claim, I started talking about brown squiggly worms, at which point I apparently lost their sympathy. It must have been a good sedative.

Regardless of the lumbar puncture I had things to do, or to have done to me, and people to see. My head was pounding and waves of nausea washed over me but I was up and off down into the bowels of the hospital for my bone scans. In an illogical way I believed that total compliance might somehow help me survive. The bone scans were slow and required total stillness. My head was taped to the table to avoid any undesirable movements. I lay there feeling sicker and sicker, counting seconds and willing time to accelerate before I needed to vomit and ruined the scans. Although so obviously necessary, I found these highly technical tests an alienating and isolating experience. What were they? How did they work? I imagined myself as a toy on a factory production line being scanned as a quality check and triggering the faulty goods alarm.

The end of the production line was the biopsy on the lump in my neck. Not high tech, just a long needle. The doctor who took it asked sympathetically which tests I'd been through that day.

'Never mind, this is the last one and it won't take long' he reassured me.

Once it was over I lay exhausted on my hospital bed. I refused to get in it, as if it were an admission of sickness. My head ached so much though, it was good to be flat. I craved the oblivion of sleep. My door opened again and a man put his head around the door. That was my first meeting with Andrew, a medical psychologist working in the cancer area, who was, over the following months, to become a valued guide, support and friend. As a psychologist myself I knew I was experiencing acute anxiety and panic attacks. I would suddenly find it difficult to breathe, as if a tight band was constricting across my chest. It wasn't just my chest constricting but also my mind. I pictured someone heating up a metal headband so that it would just fit over my forehead, and leaving it to cool so that it contracted, squeezing tighter until it could not be removed. Just as they used to make wooden barrels in years gone by, my head had become a barrel, pulled in so tightly that not a thought could escape. I was looking at myself on two levels. Half of me was objectively diagnosing myself, the other half was screaming in blind panic 'But this is happening to me, it's happening to ME.'

I had described my 'barrel' symptoms to Dr Norton, and asked if there was anyone I could talk to. To his credit Dr Norton contacted Andrew. We talked for a while until Dr Norton appeared. At this point Naomi christened him 'Ping'. He had an amazing ability to just pop up, appearing from nowhere, and disappear just as quickly. We almost expected to see a puff of smoke. 'Ping' she muttered under her breath as he happily popped back into the room with his characteristically exuberant energy.

Ping sat down in a chair and chatted to us. After a while he shifted his weight forward in the chair. His manner changed, his face becoming more formal and professional as he began to talk about the test results. Slowly and clearly he told me that the lump in my neck was not, as I had continued desperately to believe, my glandular fever biting back, but that the tumour had spread to the lymph nodes in my neck. My mind started playing with the figures that seemed to be emblazoned across it in indelible ink; 10–25%, surely this so recent news took me down to the 10%. I was angry and upset. I wanted a positive plan for the future, to look forward. A one in four chance was possible, 25% was a manageable figure, but a one in ten, that was nothing. The metal band enclosed around my head, and a further one around my chest. They squeezed and squeezed, forcing out my air, my thoughts, my being. I couldn't breathe, gulping for air as I cried hysterically.

'It's going to be all right' Naomi tried to calm me.

But it wasn't going to be all right. How could it be? I sobbed and sobbed, unable to control my shaking.

'Sorry' I blurted out, between my gulping.

'We've got plenty of time' Ping reassured me. I gradually got control of my breath and tried to focus on the figure sitting in the chair beside me.

'There is some good news as well' he continued, 'the bone scans were clear.'

So the mental calculations began again. What were my chances now? Left alone for a while I continued my hypothetical arithmetic continuously, to be interrupted a few hours later by Ping reappearing with further arbitrary data for my calculation while Naomi was trying to feed me a Thai takeaway for dinner as I lay flat on my back. I was like a baby bird trying to squawk but getting another mouthful of worm every time I opened my beak. Every time I tried to ask a question I got another forkful of stir-fried beef. The bone marrow biopsy and spinal fluid test results were OK.

The following day I was allowed home. I had been in the hospital less than 48 hours but it had felt like a whole other lifetime. I lay flat on my back for several days. The spinal fluid had leaked a little and the headaches persisted for over a week. Every time I put the 'phone down it rang, reverberating through my sore head. The doorbell went constantly. I felt like I was holding court from my bed. So many friends were wanting to do anything they could to help me. I wanted to be able to help myself. Cancer is so terrifying because it is so disempowering. I told the same story over and over again in endless repetition. I joked that I should just leave a recorded message on the answer machine, or make a general handout. In truth it had all got too much for me; the more I repeated the events of the last few days the more real it became. Naomi joined forces with the answer phone to screen calls. Everyone had different advice: dietary changes, Chinese mushrooms, beetroot juice was a big favourite, and even jumping in a particular lagoon with supposedly 'healing properties'. I couldn't concentrate. My mind was full of thoughts about the next step I was facing – chemotherapy.

Clive Sinclair

The machine is my shepherd. It leads me through the valley of the shadow of death. It judges my kidneys and finds them wanting. Even though I am full of guilt, it forgives me. It effortlessly draws the poisons from my body, it cleanses me of sin.

This ironic psalm to a mechanical god, the renal dialysis machine, is the core of Clive Sinclair's autobiographical story.

A prize-winning novelist and short-story writer, Sinclair was 43 years old when he was diagnosed as suffering from a hereditary polycystic kidney disease. Three years later he was in end-stage renal failure, and had to undergo dialysis for a year. In 1995 he had a successful kidney transplant.

Sinclair is the author of five novels, and three collections of stories, including *Blood Libels* (1985), *The Lady with the Laptop* (1996) – which won PEN Silver Pen Award – *A Soap Opera From Hell* (1998) and *Meet the Wife* (2002). His first book of stories, *Hearts of Gold*, won the Somerset Maugham Award. From 1983 to 1987 he was the literary editor of the London *Jewish Chronicle*.

His account of his renal dialysis is wry and sardonic, but also poignant. Its motif is the predicament of being a patient in a modern high-tech hospital. Of how it feels to observe one's own body blending with a machine, while one's blood – once a secret, invisible, intimate liquid – now flows out publicly into this extra metallic organ, and then eventually back again. Lying helplessly in a hospital bed, Sinclair notes how he is now expected to behave: not as a person, but rather as a patient:

In their eyes I am not a man, I am a patient. As such I am required to be good humoured, stoical, dependent, and sexless.

My Life as a Pig

by Clive Sinclair

It is the end of the afternoon. The new arrival, a little boy clutching Captain Scarlet, takes one look at me and turns to the nurse. 'Mummy,' he says, 'is that man dead?' I perk up immediately. 'Of course I'm bloody not!' I cry. Nor am I Captain Scarlet, though my blood is having an out-of-body experience. It is being pumped out by my heart and drawn into a machine via a soft plastic tube. This is where most people with no kidneys end up. There is a variety of ailments that can get you here. I have polycystic kidney disease, formerly a killer. In fact, if it weren't for my mechanical organ, that little boy would have been dead right. Welcome to my secret life.

Other men sneak off to the apartments of their paramours to enjoy old-fashioned infidelity. I am more futuristic; on Mondays and Fridays I get intimate with a machine. Don't be fooled by the sign which says Renal Dialysis Unit, this is no medical facility. It is a bloody chamber whose woozy inhabitants recline like the denizens of an opium den, the better to indulge their most outrageous whims. It is a decadent brothel, an emporium of *fin de siècle* vices, a pit of sado-masochistic iniquity. No, my innocent friend, I am not dead, nor even sick. I am simply possessed by a depravity which, if it is not indulged at least twice a week, will surely kill me.

It is in the genes. Polycystic kidney disease was imported from Stashev, Poland, by my maternal grandfather. Three of his four children inherited the condition. Two, denied dialysis, died in the 1970s. The third, my mother, was luckier. She commenced dialysis in the mid-80s and continued with it until her death in 1993. And so, when a grim-faced specialist broke the news that I was following the family tradition, it wasn't exactly a shock. That was some years ago. The information made surprisingly little difference; at least it didn't until last summer, when my normal life came to an end.

In September, having been informed that my kidneys had finally collected their marching orders, I was sent to see Mr T, a surgeon at the Lister Hospital in S—. The waiting room was full of fellow sufferers. There was an old couple

I recognized from last week's clinic calmly browsing through the *Reader's Digest* while some younger counterparts seemed more distraught. The woman, an attractive blonde, clutched her husband's hand; her face was white and she was trembling. 'Are you here for treatment?' asked a nurse. The woman nodded. 'My wife is very nervous,' added her husband, whereupon the woman began to weep.

A doctor approached me. He wore thick glasses, and he had a very loud voice. 'Ah, Mr Sinclair,' he said, so that the whole neighbourhood could hear, 'you are in end-stage kidney failure, and you have been thinking about what form of dialysis you prefer. Is that right?' As it happened, he was wrong. For the past week I'd been trying to evade the subject altogether, assisted, it must be said, by the hospital's inefficiency. 'Hasn't anyone from the unit contacted you?' he enquired. I shook my head. He summoned a nurse. 'Right,' she said, 'follow me.'

There are two types of dialysis available: the familiar, vampiristic haemo-dialysis and the more mysterious CAPD (an acronym for continuous ambu-latory peritoneal dialysis). The latter sounds much less fearful, less traumatic, and can be done at home; but it does require the dialysand to infuse a special fluid, which absorbs excess waste and water, into the peritoneal cavity four times every day. Alas, this isn't done via the bellybutton.

The nurse led me to a large room. In its centre, hanging like a grotesque fashion accessory, was something that resembled a flak jacket with a six-inch plastic umbilical cord. The nurse tweaked it. 'This is the catheter through which the fluid is admitted and expelled,' she explained. 'It's Mr T's job to insert it in your abdomen.' I tried on the jacket and peered in the mirror. It did not suit me. I definitely did not like the idea of sprouting a second omphalos in my mid-forties. Presumably I'd also sound like the kitchen sink, with two litres of that special fluid continually on the move in my belly. The nurse handed me a booklet entitled *Peritoneal Dialysis*. It had a rainbow on the cover. Inside were drawings of a man with various bags attached to the catheter. He was naked, but had no genitals. Were the anonymous authors sending me a subliminal message?

We were talking big issues here, so I decided not to be shy. 'How about my sex life?' I asked.

'There's usually some embarrassment at first,' admitted the nurse, 'but if your partner is willing there's no reason why you shouldn't continue to enjoy normal sexual relations.' My late wife would have been game, I am sure, but what is a complete stranger going to think when I start to look shifty on our first night and whisper, 'Before I take off my clothes there's something that you ought to know about me . . .' I remembered that the sight of David Bowie sans *pupik* in *The Man Who Fell to Earth* made me want to throw up. How could I expect a girl not to faint if she witnessed something even more grotesque?

Of course there were other considerations beside getting laid, but this isn't *War and Peace*, so we'll stick to the point. I was asking the nurse if there was any evidence that the alternative method – haemodialysis – caused impotence, when Mr T's secretary appeared and beckoned me to follow her to the surgeon's lair.

Mr T was invisible, being flanked by two opaque flunkies, one of whom I had already met. All I could hear was a plummy voice that sounded on the point of demanding a Pimms No. 1. No one looked at me, let alone offered a word of greeting. The secretary and the nurse, who had tagged along, stood in front of the door, as if to prevent my escape. I sat down and tried to convert my apprehension into aggression. Eventually, after ten minutes or so, the bit-players parted like the Red Sea and the newly revealed Mr T said, as if to no one in particular: 'All right, roll up your sleeves and lie on the couch.'

'Are you talking to me?' I said, trying to pitch the sound somewhere between naivety and fury.

'Come to the couch, *please*,' said Mr T.

At first things went swimmingly. 'No problems here,' said Mr T as he pumped up my left arm and examined the veins. If I plumped for haemodialysis he would have to effect a subcutaneous connection between an artery and one of those unproblematic veins. The resulting confluence being called a 'fistula' or a 'Cimino' (after the clinician who developed the procedure, rather than the bloodthirsty film director). Incidentally, Mr T's comment was not directed at me, but at his sidekicks (neither was introduced, so I'll call them 'Glasses' and 'Moustache').

The latter, Moustache, then ordered me to unbutton my shirt and loosen my trousers. I undid the belt. It didn't suffice. 'We need to feel around your groin,' said Moustache, as he exposed his cousin, Pubic Hair. 'A big cough, please,' said Mr T, as he began to palpate Tierra del Fuego. 'Cough again,' he continued. Before long it sounded like Franz Kafka was in the room. 'What do you make of this?' he asked Glasses. 'A bit facel-vega, don't you think?'

Facel-vega? Had I heard right? Isn't that a make of car?

'Definitely,' agreed Glasses.

I was asked to stand up. 'Lower your trousers a bit more,' said Moustache. I dropped them a couple of inches. 'No,' said Moustache, 'let go of them altogether.' I was particularly reluctant to release them, although they were covering nothing. But I had no choice. My penultimate line of defence crumpled to the floor. I thanked God that I was wearing my Greenpeace boxers with their discreet dolphin motif, rather than my brazen Popeye shorts with the cartoon characters and the hearts. Not for long. With a single tug, Moustache removed them and Mr T grabbed my naked balls and ordered me to cough yet again. 'Yes,' he said, 'definitely facel-vega.'

I was thinking three things. 1) That I didn't like this Sloane Ranger fondling my balls as if they were kiwi fruit in a supermarket. 2) That he had discovered some further, dread disease in the body politic, such that my polycystic kidneys will be looked upon as old and trusted friends. 3) That the nurse, with whom I was discussing my sex life a few minutes before, would now be of the opinion that I actually had nothing to lose.

'No doubt about it,' echoed Moustache, 'it's facel-vega.' I can take no more.
'Would you mind translating?' I said.

'In good time,' replied Mr T, still holding my balls. Eventually he permitted me to pull up my trousers, informing me that I had the beginnings of an inguinal hernia, which would have to be repaired with extra surgery if I opted for CAPD. That settled it. 'In that case I'll go for the haemodialysis,' I said.

'I'm beginning to feel like a waiter taking orders,' complained Mr T, wittily, 'with patients saying they'll take this, or don't feel like that.'

'Better a waiter than the main course,' I replied.

And so the fistula was made. There were three of us in the ward who had all survived the operation. We shuffled around, our wounded arms forming right angles, outstretched and wrapped in white mufflers. We resembled a trio of trainee falconers awaiting the return of our absconding birds.

The doctor at the next renal clinic confirmed that Mr T had done an excellent job. The fistula was working well. When touched it buzzed like a live wire. In the trade this was known as a thrill. I had never seen this doctor before. He was wearing a black tie. Dr V (a name tag was attached to his stethoscope) was obviously not big on tact. None the less, I attempted to make contact. He had a pronounced Spanish accent. 'Where are you from?' I enquired.

'Colombia,' he replied, 'in South America.'

'I know where Colombia is,' I said.

'Oh,' he said, 'most people don't.'

I began to wonder if this man could be an ersatz doctor, an impostor, an out-of-work actor who had wandered in off the streets. Especially when he made the dread pronouncement: 'You must commence dialysis as soon as possible.'

The first time is like losing your virginity. 'You will feel a little prick,' said the nurse as she drove in the needle.

'Don't worry,' I replied, 'I feel one already.' Needless to say, the nurses don't regard themselves as sex objects. To them the dialysis unit is utterly devoid of erotica, merely a place of work. They obviously want me to stay well, but aren't particularly interested in the characteristics that usually attach themselves to that condition. In their eyes I am not a man, I am a patient. As such I am required to be good humoured, stoical, dependent, and sexless; *Homus dunkerqus*.

And so it happens, on occasion, when I am having the needles removed at the end of my trial, I feel soft flesh nesting in my cupped hand and realize that I am holding the left breast of my saviour. I don't blame the nurses for regarding me as an *it* rather than a *thou*, I recognize that they require strategies to retain their equilibrium, just as I do. I understand why they prefer to keep their real lives under wraps, but must advise them that their uniforms are much more charitable with their underwear. Like Andre Agassi's shorts at Wimbledon these tend to transparency. You can find out a lot of things about a person by studying their knickers, which I often do as the hours drag by. Forgive me, my sisters of mercy, forgive my voyeuristic impulses, forgive my petty attempt to reassert my masculinity, to convince myself – if not the little boy with Captain Scarlet – that there's life in the old dog.

There is just one escape from my predicament (excluding death): a transplant. At present the only available donors are the brain-dead, a much smaller proportion of the population than you'd expect. So I'm investing my hopes in Astrid. Astrid is a pig. Hitherto any xenotransplantations would have been negated by a protein called 'complement'. This is the immigration official from hell, the body's own Dirty Harry, conditioned to track down every scrap of foreign tissue and blow it away with the equivalent of a .45 magnum. Astrid, however, has been genetically engineered to develop hearts and kidneys that will sweet-talk and switch off this rejection process. She is already the matriarch of three generations, hundreds of descendants, all running around with what are, in effect, human organs. I'd be proud to call her Mum.

I am well aware that some have ethical problems with this use of animals. Supposing I decide to remarry (about as likely as a transplant). I can't quite picture my bride-to-be, but I can see my prospective mother-in-law with frightening clarity.

'Well,' she'll ask, 'is he Jewish?'

To which her daughter will reply, 'Most of him.'

Whereupon she'll want to know which bit isn't. So I'll tell her. The vision of grandchildren with trotters and curly tails will surely prove too much for the poor woman. 'Oy!' she'll wail. 'Fetch the rabbi!' Actually she need not torture herself; the former chief rabbi has already given his blessing to such transgenic procedures, as has a senior Muslim cleric. So long as the unkosher flesh is not ingested, the animal isn't forbidden; anyway, both religions regard the preservation of life as the most pressing and sacred of duties.

A more radical alternative is offered by David Cronenberg – an aficionado of metamorphosis – in his horror flick, *Shivers*. 'What we were trying to find was an alternative to organ transplant,' explains a scientist while chewing on a gerkin. '. . . To you organ transplant is just yesterday's kishkas, right? Look, you got man, right? And you got parasites that live in, on, or around man, right? So. Why not, why not breed a parasite that can do something useful, huh? A parasite that can take over the function of a human organ. For example; you breed a parasite that you implant in the human body cavity. It locks into the circulatory system, and it filters the blood just like a kidney does. So it takes a little blood for itself once in a while, what do you care? I mean, you've got enough, you can afford to be generous, huh? . . . Look, you got a guy with a bad kidney, right, and you put the bug in. The bug goes to work on the kidney – dissolves it – the body assimilates it. Now, what have you got? You've got a perfectly good parasite where you used to have a rotten kidney, right?' Needless to say, the project goes horribly wrong; is sabotaged at the outset by the explicator's partner, who has an entirely different agenda. His aim is to free the body from the mind, the id from the ego. Instead of new kidneys or new hearts his victims end up with uncontrollable urges to fornicate.

Lest you begin to believe that I have been thus doctored, I shall forget about sex, and reveal my serious side. For instance, when the nurse runs tubes around my left arm, as she connects me to the machine, I recall the days before my bar mitzvah, when I was compelled to wrap phylacteries around that same limb, thereby dedicating my heart to God. What I didn't know then was that God was equally keen on kidneys. Recently a well-educated friend pointed out that in biblical times the kidney was regarded as the seat of guilt and, as such, was often the subject of divine scrutiny. I consulted the Good Book, and saw that he was right. 'O let the wickedness of the wicked come to an end; but establish the just,' saith David the psalmist. 'For the righteous God trieth the hearts and kidneys.' Later he adds, for good measure, 'The darkness and the light are both alike to thee. Thou has possessed my kidneys.' Jeremiah is even blunter: 'But, O Lord of hosts, that judgest righteously, that triest the kidneys and the heart, let me see thy vengeance.'

Most would regard this as an abstract concept, certainly nothing to worry about in this life. Not me. My heart is tried periodically with an ECG, my kidneys tested week in week out. I may pretend that the hospital is a whore-house devoted to the pleasure principle, but I know that it is really a place of severe judgements. I go there because of my guilt. If modern philosophers are correct and there is no distinction between mind and body, then this guilt is a material thing, nameable and quantifiable. There is my creatinine, five times higher than normal, and my urea, a mere three times over the top. What has led to this guilty state I really do not know. Perhaps I am being punished for an unpardonable iniquity committed by a distant ancestor. Anyway, there is irony in an atheist (albeit a Jewish one) who has always regarded God as immaterial suddenly finding himself subject to a machine with divine attributes. Surely our nonverbal communication is a form of prayer.

The machine is my shepherd. It leads me through the valley of the shadow of death. It judges my kidneys and finds them wanting. Even though I am full of guilt, it forgives me. It effortlessly draws the poisons from my body, it cleanses me of sin. At the end of my three hours I am ready to return to the world, shriven, my soul like a newly laundered sheet. 'I'm done!' I cry. One of the vestal virgins approaches. She releases me, then unhooks a transparent bag, bulging with my filtered venom, and drops it in the bin.

Suddenly, as if in a vision, I recognize my crime. I am here because I am a writer. The entire process is but a metaphor for my craft. For creatinine read creativity. It builds up within, like poison, until I can do nothing but discharge it. Out it flows, lava from Mt Ego, streaming across the page. And where do these outpourings end up? Like my other toxins, in the bin. Poetic justice, you might say.

W Somerset Maugham

A sanatorium, somewhere in the north of Scotland. A small, timeless world of tuber-cular patients. Waiting to live, or to die.

Using a literary device similar to Thomas Mann's *The Magic Mountain*, Maugham describes how the patients in *Sanatorium* live in their own community of suffering, their own tiny world within a world, cut off from the usual concerns of everyday life. His story recalls an era when tuberculosis – like cancer and other chronic disease today – had no chemical 'quick fix'. A time when there was not yet any pharmaceutical 'magic bullet' that could destroy the bacteria of the killer disease, and restore the patient to health. Instead – in addition to their largely ineffective remedies – all the doctors had to rely on were the more ancient sources of healing: Nature and Time, and the patient's body and will. Rest, 'fresh air', a good diet, moderate exercise, mountain views and lots of bright sunlight were all considered a crucial part of the cure.

W Somerset Maugham was one of the most famous short-story writers of the 20th century. He was also a novelist, essayist, playwright and travel writer. In 1897, he qualified as a doctor at St Thomas' Hospital in London, and for a while practised in the slums of London's East End – before finally giving up medicine for literature. Although his medical career was short-lived, he drew on these early experiences for two of his most famous novels: *Liza of Lambeth* (1897) and *Of Human Bondage* (1915).

Sanatorium

by W Somerset Maugham

For the first six weeks that Ashenden was at the sanatorium he stayed in bed. He saw nobody but the doctor who visited him morning and evening, the nurses who looked after him and the maid who brought him his meals. He had contracted tuberculosis of the lungs and since at the time there were reasons that made it difficult for him to go to Switzerland the specialist he saw in London had sent him up to a sanatorium in the north of Scotland. At last the day came that he had been patiently looking forward to when the doctor told him he could get up; and in the afternoon his nurse, having helped him to dress, took him down to the verandah, placed cushions behind him, wrapped him up in rugs and left him to enjoy the sun that was streaming down from a cloudless sky. It was mid-winter. The sanatorium stood on the top of a hill and from it you had a spacious view of the snow-clad country. There were people lying all along the verandah in deckchairs, some chatting with their neighbours and some reading. Every now and then one would have a fit of coughing and you noticed that at the end of it he looked anxiously at his handkerchief. Before the nurse left Ashenden she turned with a kind of professional briskness to the man who was lying in the next chair.

'I want to introduce Mr. Ashenden to you,' she said. And then to Ashenden: 'This is Mr. McLeod. He and Mr. Campbell have been here longer than anyone else.'

On the other side of Ashenden was lying a pretty girl, with red hair and bright blue eyes; she had on no make-up, but her lips were very red and the colour on her cheeks was high. It emphasised the astonishing whiteness of her skin. It was lovely even when you realised that its delicate texture was due to illness. She wore a fur coat and was wrapped up in rugs, so that you could see nothing of her body, but her face was extremely thin, so thin that it made her nose, which wasn't really large, look a trifle prominent. She gave Ashenden a friendly look, but did not speak, and Ashenden, feeling rather shy among all those strange people, waited to be spoken to.

'First time they've let you get up, is it?' said McLeod.

'Yes.'

'Where's your room?'

Ashenden told him.

'Small. I know every room in the place. I've been here for seventeen years. I've got the best room here and so I damned well ought to have. Campbell's been trying to get me out of it, he wants it himself, but I'm not going to budge; I've got a right to it, I came here six months before he did.'

McLeod, lying there, gave you the impression that he was immensely tall; his skin was stretched tight over his bones, his cheeks and temples hollow, so that you could see the formation of his skull under it; and in that emaciated face, with its great bony nose, the eyes were preternaturally large.

'Seventeen years is a long time,' said Ashenden, because he could think of nothing else to say.

'Time passes very quickly. I like it here. At first, after a year or two, I went away in the summer, but I don't any more. It's my home now. I've got a brother and two sisters; but they're married and now they've got families; they don't want me. When you've been here a few years and you go back to ordinary life, you feel a bit out of it, you know. Your pals have gone their own ways and you've got nothing in common with them any more. It all seems an awful rush. Much ado about nothing, that's what it is. It's noisy and stuffy. No, one's better off here. I shan't stir again till they carry me out feet first in my coffin.'

The specialist had told Ashenden that if he took care of himself for a reasonable time he would get well, and he looked at McLeod with curiosity.

'What do you do with yourself all day long?' he asked.

'Do? Having T.B. is a whole time job, my boy. There's my temperature to take and then I weigh myself. I don't hurry over my dressing. I have breakfast, I read the papers and go for a walk. Then I have my rest. I lunch and play bridge. I have another rest and then I dine. I play a bit more bridge and I go to bed. They've got quite a decent library here, we get all the new books, but I don't really have much time for reading. I talk to people. You meet all sorts here, you know. They come and they go. Sometimes they go because they think they're cured, but a lot of them come back, and sometimes they go because they die. I've seen a lot of people out and before I go I expect to see a lot more.'

The girl sitting on Ashenden's other side suddenly spoke.

'I should tell you that few persons can get a heartier laugh out of a hearse than Mr. McLeod,' she said.

McLeod chuckled.

'I don't know about that, but it wouldn't be human nature if I didn't say to myself: Well, I'm just as glad it's him and not me they're taking for a ride.'

It occurred to him that Ashenden didn't know the pretty girl, so he introduced him.

'By the way, I don't think you've met Mr. Ashenden – Miss Bishop. She's English, but not a bad girl.'

'How long have *you* been here?' asked Ashenden.

'Only two years. This is my last winter. Dr. Lennox says I shall be all right in a few months and there's no reason why I shouldn't go home.'

'Silly, I call it,' said McLeod. 'Stay where you're well off, that's what I say.'

At that moment a man, leaning on a stick, came walking slowly along the verandah.

'Oh, look, there's Major Templeton,' said Miss Bishop, a smile lighting up her blue eyes; and then, as he came up: 'I'm glad to see you up again.'

'Oh, it was nothing. Only a bit of a cold. I'm quite all right now.'

The words were hardly out of his mouth when he began to cough. He leaned heavily on his stick. But when the attack was over he smiled gaily.

'Can't get rid of this damned cough,' he said. 'Smoking too much. Dr. Lennox says I ought to give it up, but it's no good – I can't.'

He was a tall fellow, good-looking in a slightly theatrical way, with a dusky, sallow face, fine very dark eyes and a neat black moustache. He was wearing a fur coat with an Astrakhan collar. His appearance was smart and perhaps a trifle showy. Miss Bishop made Ashenden known to him. Major Templeton said a few civil words in an easy, cordial way, and then asked the girl to go for a stroll with him; he had been ordered to walk to a certain place in the wood behind the sanatorium and back again. McLeod watched them as they sauntered off.

'I wonder if there's anything between those two,' he said. 'They do say Templeton was a devil with the girls before he got ill.'

'He doesn't look up to much in that line just now,' said Ashenden.

'You never can tell. I've seen a lot of rum things here in my day. I could tell you no end of stories if I wanted to.'

'You evidently do, so why don't you?'

McLeod grinned.

'Well, I'll tell you one. Three or four years ago there was a woman here who was pretty hot stuff. Her husband used to come and see her every other week-end, he was crazy about her, used to fly up from London; but Dr. Lennox was pretty sure she was carrying on with somebody here, but he couldn't find out who. So one night when we'd all gone to bed he had a thin coat of paint put down just outside her room and next day he had everyone's slippers examined. Neat, wasn't it? The fellow whose slippers had paint on them got the push. Dr. Lennox has to be particular, you know. He doesn't want the place to get a bad name.'

'How long has Templeton been here?'

'Three or four months. He's been in bed most of the time. He's for it all right. Ivy Bishop'll be a damned fool if she gets stuck on him. She's got a good chance of getting well. I've seen so many of them, you know, I can tell. When I look at a fellow I make up my mind at once whether he'll get well or whether he won't, and if he won't I can make a pretty shrewd guess how long he'll last. I'm very seldom mistaken. I give Templeton about two years myself.'

McLeod gave Ashenden a speculative look and Ashenden, knowing what he was thinking, though he tried to be amused, could not help feeling somewhat concerned. There was a twinkle in McLeod's eyes. He plainly knew what was passing through Ashenden's mind.

'You'll get all right. I wouldn't have mentioned it if I hadn't been pretty sure of that. I don't want Dr. Lennox to hoof me out for putting the fear of God into his bloody patients.'

Then Ashenden's nurse came to take him back to bed. Even though he had only sat out for an hour, he was tired, and was glad to find himself once more between the sheets. Dr. Lennox came in to see him in the course of the evening. He looked at his temperature chart.

'That's not so bad,' he said.

Dr. Lennox was small, brisk and genial. He was a good enough doctor, an excellent business man, and an enthusiastic fisherman. When the fishing season began he was inclined to leave the care of his patients to his assistants; the patients grumbled a little, but were glad enough to eat the young salmon he brought back to vary their meals. He was fond of talking, and now, standing at the end of Ashenden's bed, he asked him, in his broad Scots, whether he had got into conversation with any of the patients that afternoon. Ashenden told him the nurse had introduced him to McLeod. Dr. Lennox laughed.

'The oldest living inhabitant. He knows more about the sanatorium and its inmates than I do. How he gets his information I haven't an idea, but there's not a thing about the private lives of anyone under this roof that he doesn't know. There's not an old maid in the place with a keener nose for a bit of scandal. Did he tell you about Campbell?'

'He mentioned him.'

'He hates Campbell, and Campbell hates him. Funny, when you come to think of it, those two men, they've been here for seventeen years and they've got about one sound lung between them. They loathe the sight of one another. I've had to refuse to listen to the complaints about one another that they come to me with. Campbell's room is just below McLeod's and Campbell plays the fiddle. It drives McLeod wild. He says he's been listening to the same tunes for fifteen years, but Campbell says McLeod doesn't know one tune from another. McLeod wants me to stop Campbell playing, but I can't do that, he's got a perfect right to play so long as he doesn't play in the silence hours. I've offered to change McLeod's room, but he won't do that. He says Campbell only plays to drive him out of the room because it's the best in the house, and he's damned if he's going to have it. It's queer, isn't it, that two middle-aged men should think it worth while to make life hell for one another. Neither can leave the other alone. They have their meals at the same table, they play bridge together; and not a day passes without a row. Sometimes I've threatened to turn them both out if they don't behave like sensible fellows. That keeps them quiet for a bit. They don't want to go. They've been here so long, they've got no one any more who gives a damn for them, and they can't cope with the world outside.

Campbell went away for a couple of months' holiday some years ago. He came back after a week; he said he couldn't stand the racket, and the sight of so many people in the streets scared him.'

It was a strange world into which Ashenden found himself thrown when, his health gradually improving, he was able to mix with his fellow patients. One morning Dr. Lennox told him he could thenceforward lunch in the dining-room. This was a large, low room, with great window space; the windows were always wide open and on fine days the sun streamed in. There seemed to be a great many people and it took him some time to sort them out. They were of all kinds, young, middle-aged and old. There were some, like McLeod and Campbell, who had been at the sanatorium for years and expected to die there. Others had only been there for a few months. There was one middle-aged spinster called Miss Atkin who had been coming every winter for a long time and in the summer went to stay with friends and relations. She had nothing much the matter with her any more, and might just as well have stayed away altogether, but she liked the life. Her long residence had given her a sort of position, she was honorary librarian and hand in glove with the matron. She was always ready to gossip with you, but you were soon warned that every-thing you said was passed on. It was useful to Dr. Lennox to know that his patients were getting on well together and were happy, that they did nothing imprudent and followed his instructions. Little escaped Miss Atkin's sharp eyes, and from her it went to the matron and so to Dr. Lennox. Because she had been coming for so many years, she sat at the same table as McLeod and Campbell, together with an old general who had been put there on account of his rank. The table was in no way different from any other, and it was not more advantageously placed, but because the oldest residents sat there it was looked upon as the most desirable place to sit, and several elderly women were bitterly resentful because Miss Atkin, who went away for four or five months every summer, should be given a place there while they who spent the whole year in the sanatorium sat at other tables. There was an old Indian Civilian who had been at the sanatorium longer than anyone but McLeod and Campbell; he was a man who in his day had ruled a province, and he was waiting irascibly for either McLeod or Campbell to die so that he might take his place at the first table. Ashenden made the acquaintance of Campbell. He was a long, big-boned fellow with a bald head, so thin that you wondered how his limbs held together; and when he sat crumpled in an arm-chair he gave you the uncanny impression of a mannikin in a puppet-show. He was brusque, touchy and bad-tempered. The first thing he asked Ashenden was:

'Are you fond of music?'

'Yes.'

'No one here cares a damn for it. I play the violin. But if you like it, come to my room one day and I'll play to you.'

'Don't you go,' said McLeod, who heard him. 'It's torture.'

'How can you be so rude?' cried Miss Atkin. 'Mr. Campbell plays very nicely.'

'There's no one in this beastly place that knows one note from another,' said Campbell.

With a derisive chuckle McLeod walked off. Miss Atkin tried to smooth things down.

'You mustn't mind what McLeod said.'

'Oh, I don't. I'll get back on him all right.'

He played the same tune over and over again all that afternoon. McLeod banged on the floor, but Campbell went on. He sent a message by a maid to say that he had a headache and would Mr. Campbell mind not playing; Campbell replied that he had a perfect right to play and if Mr. McLeod didn't like it he could lump it. When next they met high words passed.

Ashenden was put at a table with the pretty Miss Bishop, with Templeton, and with a London man, an accountant, called Henry Chester. He was a stocky, broad-shouldered, wiry little fellow, and the last person you would ever have thought would be attacked by T.B. It had come upon him as a sudden and unexpected blow. He was a perfectly ordinary man, somewhere between thirty, and forty, married, with two children. He lived in a decent suburb. He went up to the City every morning and read the morning paper; he came down from the City every evening and read the evening paper. He had no interests except his business and his family. He liked his work; he made enough money to live in comfort, he put by a reasonable sum every year, he played golf on Saturday afternoon and on Sunday, he went every August for a three weeks' holiday to the same place on the east coast; his children would grow up and marry, then he would turn his business over to his son and retire with his wife to a little house in the country where he could potter about till death claimed him at a ripe old age. He asked nothing more from life than that, and it was a life that thousands upon thousands of his fellow-men lived with satisfaction. He was the average citizen. Then this thing happened. He had caught cold playing golf, it had gone to his chest, and he had had a cough that he couldn't shake off. He had always been strong and healthy, and had no opinion of doctors; but at last at his wife's persuasion he had consented to see one. It was a shock to him, a fearful shock, to learn that there was tubercle in both his lungs and that his only chance of life was to go immediately to a sanatorium. The specialist he saw then told him that he might be able to go back to work in a couple of years, but two years had passed and Dr. Lennox advised him not to think of it for at least a year more. He showed him the bacilli in his sputum, and in an X-ray photograph the actively-diseased patches in his lungs. He lost heart. It seemed to him a cruel and unjust trick that fate had played upon him. He could have understood it if he had led a wild life, if he had drunk too much, played around with women or kept late hours. He would have deserved it then. But he had done none of these things. It was monstrously unfair. Having no resources in himself, no interest in books, he had nothing to do but think of his health. It became an obsession. He watched his symptoms anxiously. They had to deprive him of a thermometer because he took his temperature a dozen times a day. He got it into his head that the doctors were taking his case too indifferently, and in order to force their attention used every method he could devise to make the thermometer register a temperature that would alarm; and when his tricks were foiled he grew sulky and querulous. But he was by nature a jovial, friendly creature, and when he forgot himself he talked and laughed gaily; then on a sudden he remembered that he was a sick man and you would see in his eyes the fear of death.

At the end of every month his wife came up to spend a day or two in a lodging-house near-by. Dr. Lennox did not much like the visits that relatives paid the patients, it excited and unsettled them. It was moving to see the eagerness with which Henry Chester looked forward to his wife's arrival; but it was strange to notice that once she had come he seemed less pleased than one would have expected. Mrs. Chester was a pleasant, cheerful little woman, not pretty, but neat, as commonplace as her husband, and you only had to look at her to know that she was a good wife and mother, a careful housekeeper, a nice, quiet body who did her duty and interfered with nobody. She had been quite happy in the dull, domestic life they had led for so many years, her only dissipation a visit to the pictures, her great thrill the sales in the big London shops; and it had never occurred to her that it was monotonous. It completely satisfied her. Ashenden liked her. He listened with interest while she prattled about her children and her house in the suburbs, her neighbours and her trivial occupations. On one occasion he met her in the road. Chester for some reason connected with his treatment had stayed in and she was alone. Ashenden suggested that they should walk together. They talked for a little of indifferent things. Then she suddenly asked him how he thought her husband was.

'I think he seems to be getting on all right.'

'I'm so terribly worried.'

'You must remember it's a slow, long business. One has to have patience.'

They walked on a little and then he saw she was crying.

'You mustn't be unhappy about him,' said Ashenden gently.

'Oh, you don't know what I have to put up with when I come here. I know I ought not to speak about it, but I must. I can trust you, can't I?'

'Of course.'

'I love him. I'm devoted to him. I'd do anything in the world I could for him. We've never quarrelled, we've never even differed about a single thing. He's beginning to hate me and it breaks my heart.'

'Oh, I can't believe that. Why, when you're not here he talks of you all the time. He couldn't talk more nicely. He's devoted to you.'

'Yes, that's when I'm not here. It's when I'm here, when he sees me well and strong, that it comes over him. You see, he resents it so terribly that he's ill and I'm well. He's afraid he's going to die and he hates me because I'm going to live. I have to be on my guard all the time; almost everything I say, if I speak of the children, if I speak of the future, exasperates him, and he says bitter, wounding things. When I speak of something I've had to do to the house or a servant I've had to change it irritates him beyond endurance. He complains that I treat him as if he didn't count any more. We used to be so united, and now I feel there's a great wall of antagonism between us. I know I shouldn't blame him, I know it's only his illness, he's a dear good man really, and kindness itself, normally he's the easiest man in the world to get on with; and now I simply dread coming here and I go with relief. He'd be terribly sorry if I had T.B. but I know that in his heart of hearts it would be a relief. He could forgive me, he could forgive fate, if he thought I was going to die too. Sometimes he tortures me by talking about what I shall do when he's dead, and when I get hysterical and cry out to him to stop, he says I needn't grudge him a little pleasure when he'll be dead so soon and I can go on living for years and years and have a good time. Oh, it's so frightful to think that this love we've had for one another all these years should die in this sordid, miserable way.'

Mrs. Chester sat down on a stone by the roadside and gave way to passionate weeping. Ashenden looked at her with pity, but could find nothing to say that might comfort her. What she had told him did not come quite as a surprise.

'Give me a cigarette,' she said at last. 'I mustn't let my eyes get all red and swollen, or Henry'll know I've been crying and he'll think I've had bad news about him. Is death so horrible? Do we all fear death like that?'

'I don't know,' said Ashenden.

'When my mother was dying she didn't seem to mind a bit. She knew it was coming and she even made little jokes about it. But she was an old woman.'

Mrs. Chester pulled herself together and they set off again. They walked for a while in silence.

'You won't think any the worse of Henry for what I've told you?' she said at last.

'Of course not.'

'He's been a good husband and a good father. I've never known a better man in my life. Until this illness I don't think an unkind or ungenerous thought ever passed through his head.'

The conversation left Ashenden pensive. People often said he had a low opinion of human nature. It was because he did not always judge his fellows by the usual standards. He accepted, with a smile, a tear or a shrug of the shoulders, much that filled others with dismay. It was true that you would never have expected that good-natured, commonplace little chap to harbour such bitter and unworthy thoughts; but who has ever been able to tell to what depths man may fall or to what heights rise? The fault lay in the poverty of his ideals. Henry Chester was born and bred to lead an average life, exposed to the normal vicissitudes of existence, and when an unforeseeable accident befell him he had no means of coping with it. He was like a brick made to take its place with a million others in a huge factory, but by chance with a flaw in it so that it is inadequate to its purpose. And the brick too, if it had a mind, might cry: What have I done that I cannot fulfil my modest end, but must be taken away from all these other bricks that support me and thrown on the dust-heap? It was no fault of Henry Chester's that he was incapable of the conceptions that might have enabled him to bear his calamity with resignation. It is not everyone who can find solace in art or thought. It is the tragedy of our day that these humble souls have lost their faith in God, in whom lay hope, and their belief in a resurrection that might bring them the happiness that has been denied them on earth; and have found nothing to put in their place.

There are people who say that suffering ennobles. It is not true. As a general rule it makes man petty, querulous and selfish; but here in this sanatorium there was not much suffering. In certain stages of tuberculosis the slight fever that accompanies it excites rather than depresses, so that the patient feels alert and, upborne by hope, faces the future blithely; but for all that the idea of death haunts the subconscious. It is a sardonic theme song that runs through a sprightly operetta. Now and again the gay, melodious arias, the dance measures, deviate strangely into tragic strains that throb menacingly down the nerves; the petty interests of every day, the small jealousies and trivial concerns are as nothing; pity and terror make the heart on a sudden stand still and the awfulness of death broods as the silence that precedes a tropical storm broods over the tropical jungle. After Ashenden had been for some time at the sanatorium there came a boy of twenty. He was in the navy, a sub-lieutenant in a submarine, and he had what they used to call in novels galloping consumption. He was a tall, good-looking youth, with curly brown hair, blue eyes and a very sweet smile. Ashenden saw him two or three times lying on the terrace in the sun and passed the time of day with him. He was a cheerful lad. He talked of musical shows and film stars; and he read the paper for the football results and the boxing news. Then he was put to bed and Ashenden saw him no more. His relations were sent for and in two months he was dead. He died uncomplaining. He understood what was happening to him as little as an animal. For a day or two there was the same malaise in the sanatorium as there is in a prison when a man has been hanged; and then, as though by universal consent, in obedience to an instinct of self-preservation, the boy was put out of mind: life, with its three meals a day, its golf on the miniature course, its regulated exercise, its prescribed rests, its quarrels and jealousies, its scandal-mongering and petty vexations, went on as before. Campbell, to the exasperation of McLeod, continued to play the prize-song and 'Annie Laurie' on his fiddle. McLeod continued to boast of his bridge and gossip about other people's health and morals. Miss Atkin continued to backbite. Henry Chester continued to complain that the doctors gave him insufficient attention and railed against fate because, after the model life he had led, it had played him such a dirty trick. Ashenden continued to read, and with amused tolerance to watch the vagaries of his fellow-creatures.

He became intimate with Major Templeton. Templeton was perhaps a little more than forty years of age. He had been in the Grenadier Guards, but had resigned his commission after the war. A man of ample means, he had since then devoted himself entirely to pleasure. He raced in the racing season, shot in the shooting season and hunted in the hunting season. When this was over he went to Monte Carlo. He told Ashenden of the large sums he had made and lost at baccarat. He was very fond of women and if his stories could be believed they were very fond of him. He loved good food and good drink. He knew by their first names the head waiters of every restaurant in London where you ate well. He belonged to half a dozen clubs. He had led for years a useless, selfish, worthless life, the sort of life which maybe it will be impossible for anyone to live in the future, but he had lived it without misgiving and had enjoyed it. Ashenden asked him once what he would do if he had his time over again and he answered that he would do exactly what he had done. He was an amusing talker, gay and pleasantly ironic, and he dealt with the surface of things, which was all he knew, with a light, easy and assured touch. He always had a pleasant word for the dowdy spinsters in the sanatorium and a joking one for the peppery old gentlemen, for he combined good manners with a natural kindliness. He knew his way about the superficial world of the people who have more money than they know what to do with as well as he knew his way about Mayfair. He was the kind of man who would always have been willing to take a bet, to help a friend and to give a tenner to a rogue. If he had never done much good in the world he had never done much harm. He amounted to nothing. But he was a more agreeable companion than many of more sterling character and of more admirable qualities. He was very ill now. He was dying and he knew it. He took it with the same easy, laughing nonchalance as he had taken all the rest. He'd had a thundering good time, he regretted nothing, it was rotten tough luck getting T.B. but to hell with it, no one can live for ever, and when you came to think of it, he might have been killed in the war or broken his bloody neck in a point-to-point. His principle all through life had been, when you've made a bad bet, pay up and forget about it. He'd had a good run for his money and he was ready to call it a day. It had been a damned good party while it lasted, but every party's got to come to an end, and next day it doesn't matter much if you went home with the milk or if you left while the fun was in full swing.

Of all those people in the sanatorium he was probably from the moral standpoint the least worthy, but he was the only one who genuinely accepted the inevitable with unconcern. He snapped his fingers in the face of death, and you could choose whether to call his levity unbecoming or his insouciance gallant.

The last thing that ever occurred to him when he came to the sanatorium was that he might fall more deeply in love there than he had ever done before. His amours had been numerous, but they had been light; he had been content with the politely mercenary love of chorus girls and with ephemeral unions with women of easy virtue whom he met at house parties. He had always taken care to avoid any attachment that might endanger his freedom. His only aim in life had been to get as much fun out of it as possible, and where sex was concerned he found every advantage and no inconvenience in ceaseless variety. But he liked women. Even when they were quite old he could not talk to them without

a caress in his eyes and a tenderness in his voice. He was prepared to do anything to please them. They were conscious of his interest in them and were
agreeably flattered, and they felt, quite mistakenly, that they could trust him
never to let them down. He once said a thing that Ashenden thought showed
insight:

'You know, any man can get any woman he wants if he tries hard enough,
there's nothing in that, but once he's got her, only a man who thinks the world
of women can get rid of her without humiliating her.'

It was simply from habit that he began to make love to Ivy Bishop. She
was the prettiest and the youngest girl in the sanatorium. She was in point of
fact not so young as Ashenden had first thought her, she was twenty-nine, but
for the last eight years she had been wandering from one sanatorium to
another, in Switzerland, England and Scotland, and the sheltered invalid life
had preserved her youthful appearance so that you might easily have taken her
for twenty. All she knew of the world she had learnt in these establishments,
so that she combined rather curiously extreme innocence with extreme sophis-
tication. She had seen a number of love affairs run their course. A good many
men, of various nationalities, had made love to her; she accepted their attentions
with self-possession and humour, but she had at her disposal plenty of firm-
ness when they showed an inclination to go too far. She had a force of character
unexpected in anyone who looked so flower-like and when it came to a show-
down knew how to express her meaning in plain, cool and decisive words. She
was quite ready to have a flirtation with George Templeton. It was a game
she understood, and though always charming to him, it was with a bantering
lightness that showed quite clearly that she had summed him up and had no
mind to take the affair more seriously than he did. Like Ashenden, Templeton
went to bed every evening at six and dined in his room, so that he saw Ivy only
by day. They went for little walks together, but otherwise were seldom alone.
At lunch the conversation between the four of them, Ivy, Templeton, Henry
Chester and Ashenden, was general, but it was obvious that it was for neither
of the two men that Templeton took so much trouble to be entertaining. It
seemed to Ashenden that he was ceasing to flirt with Ivy to pass the time, and
that his feeling for her was growing deeper and more sincere; but he could
not tell whether she was conscious of it nor whether it meant anything to her.
Whenever Templeton hazarded a remark that was more intimate than the
occasion warranted she countered it with an ironic one that made them all
laugh. But Templeton's laugh was rueful. He was no longer content to have her
take him as a play-boy. The more Ashenden knew Ivy Bishop the more he liked
her. There was something pathetic in her sick beauty, with that lovely transparent skin, the thin face in which the eyes were so large and so wonderfully
blue; and there was something pathetic in her plight, for like so many others in
the sanatorium she seemed to be alone in the world. Her mother led a busy
social life, her sisters were married; they took but a perfunctory interest in the
young woman from whom they had been separated now for eight years. They

corresponded, they came to see her occasionally, but there was no longer very much between them. She accepted the situation without bitterness. She was friendly with everyone and prepared always to listen with sympathy to the complaints and the distress of all and sundry. She went out of her way to be nice to Henry Chester and did what she could to cheer him.

'Well, Mr. Chester,' she said to him one day at lunch, 'it's the end of the month, your wife will be coming to-morrow. That's something to look forward to.'

'No, she's not coming this month,' he said quietly, looking down at his plate.

'Oh, I am sorry. Why not? The children are all right, aren't they?'

'Dr. Lennox thinks it's better for me that she shouldn't come.'

There was a silence. Ivy looked at him with troubled eyes.

'That's tough luck, old man,' said Templeton in his hearty way. 'Why didn't you tell Lennox to go to hell?'

'He must know best,' said Chester.

Ivy gave him another look and began to talk of something else.

Looking back, Ashenden realised that she had at once suspected the truth. For next day he happened to walk with Chester.

'I'm awfully sorry your wife isn't coming,' he said. 'You'll miss her visit dreadfully.'

'Dreadfully.'

He gave Ashenden a sidelong glance. Ashenden felt that he had something he wanted to say, but could not bring himself to say it. He gave his shoulders an angry shrug.

'It's my fault if she's not coming. I asked Lennox to write and tell her not to. I couldn't stick it any more. I spend the whole month looking forward to her coming and then when she's here I hate her. You see, I resent so awfully having this filthy disease. She's strong and well and full of beans. It maddens me when I see the pain in her eyes. What does it matter to her really? Who cares if you're ill? They pretend to care, but they're jolly glad it's you and not them. I'm a swine, aren't I?'

Ashenden remembered how Mrs. Chester had sat on a stone by the side of the road and wept.

'Aren't you afraid you'll make her very unhappy, not letting her come?'

'She must put up with that. I've got enough with my own unhappiness with-out bothering with hers.'

Ashenden did not know what to say and they walked on in silence. Suddenly Chester broke out irritably.

'It's all very well for you to be disinterested and unselfish, you're going to live. I'm going to die, and God damn it, I don't want to die. Why should I? It's not fair.'

Time passed. In a place like the sanatorium where there was little to occupy the mind it was inevitable that soon everyone should know that George Templeton was in love with Ivy Bishop. But it was not so easy to tell what her feelings were. It was plain that she liked his company, but she did not seek it, and indeed it looked as though she took pains not to be alone with him. One or two of the middle-aged ladies tried to trap her into some compromising admission, but ingenuous as she was, she was easily a match for them. She ignored their hints and met their straight questions with incredulous laughter. She succeeded in exasperating them.

'She can't be so stupid as not to see that he's mad about her.'

'She has no right to play with him like that.'

'I believe she's just as much in love with him as he is with her.'

'Dr. Lennox ought to tell her mother.'

No one was more incensed than McLeod.

'Too ridiculous. After all, nothing can come of it. He's riddled with T.B. and she's not much better.'

Campbell on the other hand was sardonic and gross.

'I'm all for their having a good time while they can. I bet there's a bit of hanky-panky going on if one only knew, and I don't blame 'em.'

'You cad,' said McLeod.

'Oh, come off it. Templeton isn't the sort of chap to play bumble-puppy bridge with a girl like that unless he's getting something out of it, and she knows a thing or two, I bet.'

Ashenden, who saw most of them, knew them better than any of the others. Templeton at last had taken him into his confidence. He was rather amused at himself.

'Rum thing at my time of life, falling in love with a decent girl. Last thing I'd ever expected of myself. And it's no good denying it, I'm in it up to the neck; if I were a well man I'd ask her to marry me to-morrow. I never knew a girl could be as nice as that. I've always thought girls, decent girls, I mean, damned bores. But she isn't a bore, she's as clever as she can stick. And pretty too. My God, what a skin! And that hair: but it isn't any of that that's bowled me over like a row of ninepins. D'you know what's got me? Damned ridiculous when you come to think of it. An old rip like me. Virtue. Makes me laugh like a hyena. Last thing I've ever wanted in a woman, but there it is, no getting away from it, she's good, and it makes me feel like a worm. Surprises you, I suppose?'

'Not a bit,' said Ashenden. 'You're not the first rake who's fallen to innocence. It's merely the sentimentality of middle age.'

'Dirty dog,' laughed Templeton.

'What does she say to it?'

'Good God, you don't suppose I've told her. I've never said a word to her that I wouldn't have said before anyone else. I may be dead in six months, and besides, what have I got to offer a girl like that?'

Ashenden by now was pretty sure that she was just as much in love with Templeton as he was with her. He had seen the flush that coloured her cheeks when Templeton came into the dining-room and he had noticed the soft glance she gave him now and then when he was not looking at her. There was a peculiar sweetness in her smile when she listened to him telling some of his old experiences. Ashenden had the impression that she basked comfortably in his love as the patients on the terrace, facing the snow, basked in the hot sunshine; but it might very well be that she was content to leave it at that, and it was certainly no business of his to tell Templeton what perhaps she had no wish that he should know.

Then an incident occurred to disturb the monotony of life. Though McLeod and Campbell were always at odds they played bridge together because, till Templeton came, they were the best players in the sanatorium. They bickered incessantly, their post-mortems were endless, but after so many years each knew the other's game perfectly and they took a keen delight in scoring off one another. As a rule Templeton refused to play with them; though a fine player he preferred to play with Ivy Bishop, and McLeod and Campbell were agreed on this, that she ruined the game. She was the kind of player who, having made a mistake that lost the rubber, would laugh and say: Well, it only made the difference of a trick. But one afternoon, since Ivy was staying in her room with a headache, Templeton consented to play with Campbell and McLeod. Ashenden was the fourth. Though it was the end of March there had been heavy snow for several days, and they played, in a verandah open on three sides to the wintry air, in fur coats and caps, with mittens on their hands. The stakes were too small for a gambler like Templeton to take the game seriously and his bidding was overbold, but he played so much better than the other three that he generally managed to make his contract or at least to come near it. But there was much doubling and redoubling. The cards ran high, so that an inordinate number of small slams were bid; it was a tempestuous game, and McLeod and Campbell lashed one another with their tongues. Half-past five arrived and the last rubber was started, for at six the bell rang to send everyone to rest. It was a hard-fought rubber, with sets on both sides, for McLeod and Campbell were opponents and each was determined that the other should not win. At ten minutes to six it was game all and the last hand was dealt. Templeton was McLeod's partner and Ashenden Campbell's. The bidding started with two clubs from McLeod; Ashenden said nothing; Templeton showed that he had substantial help, and finally McLeod called a grand slam. Campbell doubled and McLeod redoubled. Hearing this, the players at other tables who had broken off gathered round and the hands were played in deadly silence to a little crowd of onlookers. McLeod's face was white with excitement and there were beads of sweat on his brow. His hands trembled. Campbell was very grim. McLeod had to take two finesses and they both came off. He finished with a squeeze and got the last of the thirteen tricks. There was a burst of applause from the onlookers. McLeod, arrogant in victory, sprang to his feet. He shook his clenched fist at Campbell.

'Play that off on your blasted fiddle,' he shouted. 'Grand slam doubled and redoubled. I've wanted to get it all my life and now I've got it. By God. By God.'

He gasped. He staggered forward and fell across the table. A stream of blood poured from his mouth. The doctor was sent for. Attendants came. He was dead.

He was buried two days later, early in the morning so that the patients should not be disturbed by the sight of a funeral. A relation in black came from Glasgow to attend it. No one had liked him. No one regretted him. At the end of a week so far as one could tell, he was forgotten. The Indian Civilian took his place at the principal table and Campbell moved into the room he had so long wanted.

'Now we shall have peace,' said Dr. Lennox to Ashenden. 'When you think that I've had to put up with the quarrels and complaints of those two men for years and years . . . Believe me, one has to have patience to run a sanatorium. And to think that after all the trouble he's given me he had to end up like that and scare all those people out of their wits.'

'It was a bit of a shock, you know,' said Ashenden.

'He was a worthless fellow and yet some of the women have been quite upset about it. Poor little Miss Bishop cried her eyes out.'

'I suspect that she was the only who cried for him and not for herself.'

But presently it appeared that there was one person who had not forgotten him. Campbell went about like a lost dog. He wouldn't play bridge. He wouldn't talk. There was no doubt about it, he was moping for McLeod. For several days he remained in his room, having his meals brought to him, and then went to Dr. Lennox and said he didn't like it as well as his old one and wanted to be moved back. Dr. Lennox lost his temper, which he rarely did, and told him he had been pestering him to give him that room for years and now he could stay there or get out of the sanatorium. He returned to it and sat gloomily brooding.

'Why don't you play your violin?' the matron asked him at length. 'I haven't heard you play for a fortnight.'

'I haven't.'

'Why not?'

'It's no fun any more. I used to get a kick out of playing because I knew it maddened McLeod. But now nobody cares if I play or not. I shall never play again.'

Nor did he for all the rest of the time that Ashenden was at the sanatorium. It was strange, now that McLeod was dead life had lost its savour for him. With no one to quarrel with, no one to infuriate, he had lost his incentive and it was plain that it would not be long before he followed his enemy to the grave.

But on Templeton McLeod's death had another effect, and one which was soon to have unexpected consequences. He talked to Ashenden about it in his cool, detached way.

'Grand, passing out like that in his moment of triumph. I can't make out why everyone got in such a state about it. He'd been here for years, hadn't he?'

'Eighteen, I believe.'

'I wonder if it's worth it. I wonder if it's not better to have one's fling and take the consequences.'

'I suppose it depends on how much you value life.'

'But is this life?'

Ashenden had no answer. In a few months he could count on being well, but you only had to look at Templeton to know that he was not going to recover. The death-look was on his face.

'D'you know what I've done?' asked Templeton. 'I've asked Ivy to marry me.'

Ashenden was startled.

'What did she say?'

'Bless her little heart, she said it was the most ridiculous idea she'd ever heard in her life and I was crazy to think of such a thing.'

'You must admit she was right.'

'Quite. But she's going to marry me.'

'It's madness.'

'I dare say it is; but anyhow, we're going to see Lennox and ask him what he thinks about it.'

The winter had broken at last; there was still snow on the hills, but in the valleys it was melted and on the lower slopes the birch-trees were in bud all ready to burst into delicate leaf. The enchantment of spring was in the air. The sun was hot. Everyone felt alert and some felt happy. The old stagers who came only for the winter were making their plans to go south. Templeton and Ivy went to see Dr. Lennox together. They told him what they had in mind. He examined them; they were X-rayed and various tests were taken. Dr. Lennox fixed a day when he would tell them the results and in the light of this discuss their proposal. Ashenden saw them just before they went to keep the appointment. They were anxious, but did their best to make a joke of it. Dr. Lennox showed them the results of his examinations and explained to them in plain language what their condition was.

'All that's very fine and large,' said Templeton then, 'but what we want to know is whether we can get married.'

'It would be highly imprudent.'

'We know that, but does it matter?'

'And criminal if you had a child.'

'We weren't thinking of having one,' said Ivy.

'Well, then I'll tell you in very few words how the matter stands. Then you must decide for yourselves.'

Templeton gave Ivy a little smile and took her hand. The doctor went on.

'I don't think Miss Bishop will ever be strong enough to lead a normal life, but if she continues to live as she has been doing for the last eight years . . .'

'In sanatoriums?'

'Yes. There's no reason why she shouldn't live very comfortably, if not to a ripe old age, as long as any sensible person wants to live. The disease is quiescent. If she marries, if she attempts to live an ordinary life, the foci of infection may very well light up again, and what the results of that may be no one can foretell. So far as you are concerned, Templeton, I can put it even more shortly. You've seen the X-ray photos yourself. Your lungs are riddled with tubercle. If you marry you'll be dead in six months.'

'And if I don't how long can I live?'

The doctor hesitated.

'Don't be afraid. You can tell me the truth.'

'Two or three years.'

'Thank you, that's all we wanted to know.'

They went as they had come, hand in hand; Ivy was crying softly. No one knew what they said to one another; but when they came into luncheon they were radiant. They told Ashenden and Chester that they were going to be married as soon as they could get a licence. Then Ivy turned to Chester.

'I should so much like your wife to come up for my wedding. D'you think she would?'

'You're not going to be married here?'

'Yes. Our respective relations will only disapprove, so we're not going to tell them until it's all over. We shall ask Dr. Lennox to give me away.'

She looked mildly at Chester, waiting for him to speak, for he had not answered her. The other two men watched him. His voice shook a little when he spoke.

'It's very kind of you to want her. I'll write and ask her.'

When the news spread among the patients, though everyone congratulated them, most of them privately told one another that it was very injudicious; but when they learnt, as sooner or later everything that happened in the sanatorium was learnt, that Dr. Lennox had told Templeton that if he married he would be dead in six months, they were awed to silence. Even the dullest were moved at the thought of these two persons who loved one another so much that they were prepared to sacrifice their lives. A spirit of kindliness and good will descended on the sanatorium: people who hadn't been speaking spoke to one another again; others forgot for a brief space their own anxieties. Everyone seemed to share in the happiness of the happy pair. And it was not only the spring that filled those sick hearts with new hope, the great love that had taken possession of the man and the girl seemed to spread its effulgence on all that came near them. Ivy was quietly blissful; the excitement became her and she looked younger and prettier. Templeton seemed to walk on air. He laughed and joked as if he hadn't a care in the world. You would have said that he looked forward to long years of uninterrupted felicity. But one day he confided in Ashenden.

'This isn't a bad place, you know,' he said. 'Ivy's promised me that when I hand in my checks she'll come back here. She knows the people and she won't be so lonely.'

'Doctors are often mistaken,' said Ashenden. 'If you live reasonably I don't see why you shouldn't go on for a long time yet.'

'I'm only asking for three months. If I can only have that it'll be worth it.'

Mrs. Chester came up two days before the wedding. She had not seen her husband for several months and they were shy with one another. It was easy to guess that when they were alone they felt awkward and constrained. Yet

Chester did his best to shake off the depression that was now habitual and at all events at mealtimes showed himself the jolly, hearty little fellow that he must have been before he fell ill. On the eve of the wedding day they all dined together, Templeton and Ashenden both sitting up for dinner; they drank champagne and stayed up till ten joking, laughing and enjoying themselves. The wedding took place next morning in the kirk. Ashenden was best man. Everyone in the sanatorium who could stand on his feet attended it. The newly married couple were setting out by car immediately after lunch. Patients, doctors and nurses assembled to see them off. Someone had tied an old shoe on the back of the car, and as Templeton and his wife came out of the door of the sanatorium rice was flung over them. A cheer was raised as they drove away, as they drove away to love and death. The crowd separated slowly. Chester and his wife went silently side by side. After they had gone a little way he shyly took her hand. Her heart seemed to miss a beat. With a sidelong glance she saw that his eyes were wet with tears.

'Forgive me, dear,' he said. 'I've been very unkind to you.'

'I knew you didn't mean it,' she faltered.

'Yes, I did. I wanted you to suffer because I was suffering. But not any more. All this about Templeton and Ivy Bishop – I don't know how to put it, it's made me see everything differently. I don't mind dying any more. I don't think death's very important, not so important as love. And I want you to live and be happy. I don't grudge you anything any more and I don't resent anything. I'm glad now it's me that must die and not you. I wish for you everything that's good in the world. I love you.'

O Henry

Of course there was nothing the matter with me, but I was very ill.

That indignant cry is the central theme of O Henry's satirical short story – a story about hypochondria and quackery and cure. Although it is fiction, O Henry knew more about illness, medical treatment and the inside of a sanatorium than most, for his relatively short life was overshadowed by chronic alcoholism, severe ill health, financial problems and the early death of his wife.

'O Henry' was the *nom de plume* of William Sydney Porter, born in 1862 in Greenboro, North Carolina, the son of a physician. He began his working life as a licensed pharmacist, then moved to Texas to work on a sheep ranch. Later, he was a draughts-man, a bank teller and a newspaper columnist. He spent the years 1898–1901 in jail for embezzlement, during which time he began to write his short stories. During his life, O Henry wrote over 300 stories, mostly about ordinary folk in New York or Texas, often with an unexpected twist at the end. They were published in ten collections, including *Cabbages and Kings* (1904), *The Four Million* (1906) and *The Trimmed Lamp* (1907). His most famous story is probably *The Gift of the Magi* (1906), a classic story of love.

His own life was like one of his stories: bittersweet, and with an unusual twist at the end. Despite his considerable fame, when he died of cirrhosis of the liver in New York in 1910, he had only 23 cents left in his pocket.

Let Me Feel Your Pulse

by O Henry

So I went to a doctor.

'How long has it been since you took any alcohol into your system?' he asked.

Turning my head sideways, I answered, 'Oh, quite a while.'

He was a young doctor, somewhere between twenty and forty. He wore heliotrope socks, but he looked like Napoleon. I liked him immensely.

'Now,' said he, 'I am going to show you the effect of alcohol upon your circulation.' I think it was 'circulation' he said; though it may have been 'advertising.'

He bared my left arm to the elbow, brought out a bottle of whisky, and gave me a drink. He began to look more like Napoleon. I began to like him better.

Then he put a tight compress on my upper arm, stopped my pulse with the fingers, and squeezed a rubber bulb connected with an apparatus on a stand that looked like a thermometer. The mercury jumped up and down without seeming to stop anywhere; but the doctor said it registered two hundred and thirty-seven or one hundred and sixty-five or some such number.

'Now,' said he, 'you see what alcohol does to the blood-pressure.'

'It's marvellous,' said I, 'but do you think it a sufficient test? Have one on me, and let's try the other arm.' But, no!

Then he grasped my hand. I thought I was doomed and he was saying good-bye. But all he wanted to do was to jab a needle into the end of a finger and compare the red drop with a lot of fifty-cent poker chips that he had fastened to a card.

'It's the hæmoglobin test,' he explained. 'The colour of your blood is wrong.'

'Well,' said I, 'I know it should be blue; but this is a country of mix-ups. Some of my ancestors were cavaliers; but they got thick with some people on Nantucket Island, so . . .'

'I mean,' said the doctor, 'that the shade of red is too light.'

'Oh,' said I, 'it's a case of matching instead of matches.'

The doctor then pounded me severely in the region of the chest. When he did that I don't know whether he reminded me most of Napoleon or Battling or Lord Nelson. Then he looked grave and mentioned a string of grievances that the flesh is heir to – most ending in 'itis.' I immediately paid him fifteen dollars on account.

'Is or are it or some or any of them necessarily fatal?' I asked. I thought my connection with the matter justified my manifesting a certain amount of interest.

'All of them,' he answered cheerfully. 'But their progress may be arrested. With care and proper continuous treatment you may live to be eighty-five or ninety.'

I began to think of the doctor's bill. 'Eighty-five would be sufficient, I am sure,' was my comment. I paid him ten dollars more on account.

'The first thing to do,' he said, with renewed animation, 'is to find a sanatorium where you will get a complete rest for awhile, and allow your nerves to get into a better condition. I myself will go with you and select a suitable one.'

So he took me to a mad-house in the Catskills. It was on a bare mountain frequented only by infrequent frequenters. You could see nothing but stones and boulders, some patches of snow, and scattered pine trees. The young physician in charge was most agreeable. He gave me a stimulant without applying a compress to the arm. It was luncheon time, and we were invited to partake. There were about twenty inmates at little tables in the dining-room. The young physician in charge came to our table and said: 'It is a custom with our guests not to regard themselves as patients, but merely as tired ladies and gentlemen taking a rest. Whatever slight maladies they may have are *never* alluded to in conversation.'

My doctor called loudly to a waitress to bring some phosphoglycerate of lime hash, dog-bread, bromo-seltzer pancakes, and nux vomica tea for my repast. Then a sound arose like a sudden wind storm among pine trees. It was produced by every guest in the room whispering loudly, 'Neurasthenia!' – except one man with a nose, whom I distinctly heard say, 'Chronic alcoholism.' I hope to meet him again. The physician in charge turned and walked away.

An hour or so after luncheon he conducted us to the workshop – say fifty yards from the house. Thither the guests had been conducted by the physician in charge's understudy and sponge-holder – a man with feet and a blue sweater. He was so tall that I was not sure he had a face; but the Armour Packing Company would have been delighted with his hands.

'Here,' said the physician in charge, 'our guests find relaxation from past mental worries by devoting themselves to physical labour – reaction, in reality.'

There were turning-lathes, carpenter's outfits, clay-modelling tools, spinning-wheels, weaving-frames, treadmills, bass drums, enlarged-crayon-portrait apparatuses, blacksmith forges, and everything seemingly, that could interest the paying lunatic guests of a first-rate sanatorium.

'The lady making mud-pies in the corner,' whispered the physician in charge, 'is no other than – Lula Lulington, the authoress of the novel entitled *Why Love*

Loves. What she is doing now is simply to rest her mind after performing that piece of work.'

I had seen the book. 'Why doesn't she do it by writing another one instead?' I asked.

As you see, I wasn't as far gone as they thought I was.

'The gentleman pouring water through the funnel,' continued the physician in charge, 'is a Wall Street broker broken down from overwork.'

I buttoned my coat.

Others, he pointed out, were architects playing with Noah's arks, ministers reading Darwin's *Theory of Evolution*, lawyers sawing wood, tired-out society ladies talking Ibsen to the blue-sweatered sponge-holder, a neurotic millionaire lying asleep on the floor, and a prominent artist drawing a little red wagon around the room.

'You look pretty strong,' said the physician in charge to me. 'I think the best mental relaxation for you would be throwing small boulders over the mountain-side and then bringing them up again.'

I was a hundred yards away before my doctor overtook me.

'What's the matter?' he asked.

'The matter is,' said I, 'that there are no aeroplanes handy. So I am going to merrily and hastily jog the foot-pathway to yon station and catch the first unlimited-soft-coal express back to town.'

'Well,' said the doctor, 'perhaps you are right. This seems hardly the place suitable for you. But what you need is rest – absolute rest and exercise.'

That night I went to an hotel in the city, and said to the clerk: 'What I need is absolute rest and exercise. Can you give me a room with one of those tall folding-beds in it, and a relay of bell-boys to work it up and down while I rest?'

The clerk rubbed a speck off one of his finger-nails and glanced sideways at a tall man in a white hat sitting in the lobby. That man came over and asked me politely if I had seen the shrubbery at the west entrance. I had not, so he showed it to me and then looked me over.

'I thought you had 'em,' he said, not unkindly, 'but I guess you're all right. You'd better go see a doctor, old man.'

A week afterward my doctor tested my blood-pressure again without the preliminary stimulant. He looked to me a little less like Napoleon. And his socks were of a shade of tan that did not appeal to me.

'What you need,' he decided, 'is sea air and companionship.'

'Would a mermaid . . .' I began; but he slipped on his professional manner.

'I myself,' he said, 'will take you to the Hotel Bonair off the coast of Long Island and see that you get in good shape. It is a quiet, comfortable resort where you will soon recuperate.'

The Hotel Bonair proved to be a nine-hundred room fashionable hostelry on an island off the main shore. Everybody who did not dress for dinner was shoved into a side dining-room and given only a terrapin and champagne table d'hôte. The bay was a great stamping-ground for wealthy yachtsmen. The *Corsair* anchored there the day we arrived. I saw Mr. Morgan standing on deck eating a cheese sandwich and gazing longingly at the hotel. Still, it was a very inexpensive place. Nobody could afford to pay their prices. When you went away you simply left your baggage, stole a skiff, and beat it for the mainland in the night.

When I had been there one day I got a pad of monogrammed telegraph blanks at the clerk's desk and began to wire to all my friends for get-away money. My doctor and I played one game of croquet on the golf links and went to sleep on the lawn.

When we got back to town a thought seemed to occur to him suddenly. 'By the way,' he asked, 'how do you feel?'

'Relieved of very much,' I replied.

Now a consulting physician is different. He isn't exactly sure whether he is to be paid or not, and this uncertainty ensures you either the most careful or the most careless attention. My doctor took me to see a consulting physician. He made a poor guess and gave me careful attention. I liked him immensely. He put me through some co-ordination exercises.

'Have you a pain in the back of your head?' he asked. I told him I had not.

'Shut your eyes,' he ordered, 'put your feet close together, and jump backwards as far as you can.'

I was always a good backward jumper with my eyes shut, so I obeyed. My head struck the edge of the bathroom door, which had been left open and was only three feet away. The doctor was very sorry. He had overlooked the fact that the door was open. He closed it.

'Now touch your nose with your right forefinger,' he said.

'Where is it?' I asked.

'On your face,' said he.

'I mean my right forefinger,' I explained.

'Oh, excuse me,' said he. He reopened the bathroom door, and I took my finger out of the crack of it. After I had performed the marvellous digito-nasal feat I said:

'I do not wish to deceive you as to symptoms, doctor; I really have something like a pain in the back of my head.' He ignored the symptom and examined my heart carefully with a latest-popular-air-penny-in-the-slot ear-trumpet. I felt like a ballad.

'Now,' he said, 'gallop like a horse for about five minutes around the room.'

I gave the best imitation I could of a disqualified Percheron being led out of Madison Square Garden. Then, without dropping in a penny, he listened to my chest again.

'No glanders in our family, Doc,' I said.

The consulting physician held up his forefinger within three inches of my nose. 'Look at my finger,' he commanded.

'Did you ever try Pears' . . .' I began; but he went on with his test rapidly.

'Now look across the bay. At my finger. Across the bay. At my finger. At my finger. Across the bay. Across the bay. At my finger. Across the bay.' This for about three minutes.

He explained that this was a test of the action of the brain. It seemed easy to me. I never once mistook his finger for the bay. I'll bet that if he had used the phrases: 'Gaze, as it were, unpreoccupied, outward – or rather laterally – in the direction of the horizon, underlaid, so to speak, with the adjacent fluid inlet,' and 'Now, returning – or rather, in a manner, withdrawing your attention, bestow it upon my upraised digit' – I'll bet, I say, that Harry James himself could have passed the examination.

After asking me if I had ever had a grand uncle with curvature of the spine or a cousin with swelled ankles, the two doctors retired to the bathroom and sat on the edge of the bath tub for their consultation. I ate an apple, and gazed first at my finger and then across the bay.

The doctors came out looking grave. More: they looked tombstones and Tennessee-papers-please-copy. They wrote out a diet list to which I was to be restricted. It had everything that I had ever heard of to eat on it, except snails. And I never eat a snail unless it overtakes me and bites me first.

'You must follow this diet strictly,' said the doctors.

'I'd follow it a mile if I could get one-tenth of what's on it,' I answered.

'Of next importance,' they went on, 'is outdoor air and exercise. And here is a prescription that will be of great benefit to you.'

Then all of us took something. They took their hats, and I took my departure.

I went to a druggist and showed him the prescription.

'It will be $2.87 for an ounce bottle,' he said.

'Will you give me a piece of your wrapping cord?' said I.

I made a hole in the prescription, ran the cord through it, tied it around my neck, and tucked it inside. All of us have a little superstition, and mine runs to a confidence in amulets.

Of course there was nothing the matter with me, but I was very ill. I couldn't work, sleep, eat, or bowl. The only way I could get any sympathy was to go without shaving for four days. Even then somebody would say: 'Old man, you look as hardy as a pine-knot. Been up for a jaunt in the Maine woods, eh?'

Then, suddenly, I remembered that I must have outdoor air and exercise. So I went down South to John's. John is an approximate relative by verdict of a preacher standing with a little book in his hands in a bower of chrysanthemums while a hundred thousand people looked on. John has a country house seven miles from Pineville. It is at an altitude and on the Blue Ridge Mountains in a state too dignified to be dragged into this controversy. John is mica, which is more valuable and clearer than gold.

He met me at Pineville, and we took the trolley car to his home. It is a big neighbourless cottage on a hill surrounded by a hundred mountains. We got off at his little private station, where John's family and Amaryllis met and greeted us. Amaryllis looked at me a trifle anxiously.

A rabbit came bounding across the hill between us and the house. I threw down my suit-case and pursued it hot-foot. After I had run twenty yards and seen it disappear, I sat down on the grass and wept disconsolately.

'I can't catch a rabbit any more,' I sobbed. 'I'm of no further use in the world. I may as well be dead.'

'Oh, what is it – what is it, Brother John?' I heard Amaryllis say.

'Nerves a little unstrung,' said John in his calm way. 'Don't worry. Get up, you rabbit-chaser, and come on to the house before the biscuits get cold.' It was about twilight, and the mountains came up nobly to Miss Murfree's descriptions of them.

Soon after dinner I announced that I believed I could sleep for a year or two, including legal holidays. So I was shown to a room as big and cool as a flower garden, where there was a bed as broad as a lawn. Soon afterward the remainder of the household retired, and then there fell upon the land a silence.

I had not heard a silence before in years. It was absolute. I raised myself on my elbow and listened to it. Sleep! I thought that if I only could hear a star twinkle or a blade of grass sharpen itself I could compose myself to rest. I thought once that I heard a sound like the sail of a catboat flapping as it veered about in a breeze, but I decided that it was probably only a tack in the carpet. Still I listened.

Suddenly some belated little bird alighted upon the window-sill, and, in what he no doubt considered sleepy tones, enunciated the noise generally translated as 'cheep!'

I leaped into the air.

'Hey! what's the matter down there?' called John from his room above mine.

'Oh, nothing,' I answered, 'except that I accidentally bumped my head against the ceiling.'

The next morning I went out on the porch and looked at the mountains. There were forty-seven of them in sight. I shuddered, went into the big hall sitting-room of the house, selected *Pancoast's Family Practice of Medicine* from a bookcase, and began to read. John came in, took the book away from me, and led me outside. He has a farm of three hundred acres furnished with the usual complement of barns, mules, peasantry, and harrows with three front teeth broken off. I had seen such things in my childhood, and my heart began to sink.

Then John spoke of alfalfa, and I brightened at once. 'Oh, yes,' said I, 'wasn't she in the chorus of – let's see . . .'

'Green, you know,' said John, 'and tender, and you plough it under after the first season.'

'I know,' said I, 'and the grass grows over her.'

'Right,' said John. 'You know something about farming, after all.'

'I know something of some farmers,' said I, 'and a sure scythe will mow them down some day.'

On the way back to the house a beautiful and inexplicable creature walked across our path. I stopped irresistibly fascinated, gazing at it. John waited patiently, smoking his cigarette. He is a modern farmer. After ten minutes he said: 'Are you going to stand there looking at that chicken all day? Breakfast is nearly ready.'

'A chicken?' said I.

'A White Orpington hen, if you want to particularize.'

'A White Orpington hen?' I repeated, with intense interest. The fowl walked slowly away with graceful dignity, and I followed like a child after the Pied Piper. Five minutes more were allowed me by John, and then he took me by the sleeve and conducted me to breakfast.

After I had been there a week I began to grow alarmed. I was sleeping and eating well and actually beginning to enjoy life. For a man in my desperate condition that would never do. So I sneaked down to the trolley-station, took the car for Pineville, and went to see one of the best physicians in town. By this time I knew exactly what to do when I needed medical treatment. I hung my hat on the back of a chair, and said rapidly:

'Doctor, I have cirrhosis of the heart, indurated arteries, neurasthenia, neuritis, acute indigestion, and convalescence. I am going to live on a strict diet. I shall also take a tepid bath at night and a cold one in the morning. I shall endeavour to be cheerful, and fix my mind on pleasant subjects. In the way of drugs I intend to take a phosphorus pill three times a day, preferably after meals, and a tonic composed of the tinctures of gentian, cinchona, calisaya, and cardamom compound. Into each tablespoonful of this I shall mix tincture of nux vomica, beginning with one drop and increasing it a drop each day until the maximum dose is reached. I shall drop this with a medicine-dropper, which can be procured at a trifling cost at any pharmacy. Good morning.'

I took my hat and walked out. After I had closed the door I remembered something that I had forgotten to say. I opened it again. The doctor had not moved from where he had been sitting, but he gave a slightly nervous start when he saw me again.

'I forgot to mention,' said I, 'that I shall also take absolute rest and exercise.'

After this consultation I felt much better. The re-establishing in my mind of the fact that I was hopelessly ill gave me so much satisfaction that I almost became gloomy again. There is nothing more alarming to a neurasthenic than to feel himself growing well and cheerful.

John looked after me carefully. After I had evinced so much interest in his White Orpington chicken he tried his best to divert my mind, and was particular to lock his hen house of nights. Gradually the tonic mountain air, the wholesome food, and the daily walks among the hills so alleviated my malady that I became utterly wretched and despondent. I heard of a country doctor who lived in the mountains near-by. I went to see him and told him the whole story. He was a grey-bearded man with clear, blue, wrinkled eyes, in a home-made suit of grey jeans.

In order to save time I diagnosed my case, touched my nose with my right forefinger, struck myself below the knee to make my foot kick, sounded my chest, stuck out my tongue, and asked him the price of cemetery lots in Pineville.

He lit his pipe and looked at me for about three minutes. 'Brother,' he said, after awhile, 'you are in a mighty bad way. There's a chance for you to pull through, but it's a mighty slim one.'

'What can it be?' I asked eagerly. 'I have taken arsenic and gold, phosphorus, exercise, nux vomica, hydrotherapeutic baths, rest, excitement, codein, and aromatic spirits of ammonia. Is there anything left in the pharmacopœia?'

'Somewhere in these mountains,' said the doctor, 'there's a plant growing – a flowering plant that'll cure you, and it's about the only thing that will. It's of a kind that's as old as the world; but of late it's powerful scarce and hard to find. You and I will have to hunt it up. I'm not engaged in active practice now; I'm getting along in years; but I'll take your case. You'll have to come every day in the afternoon and help me hunt for this plant till we find it. The city doctors may know a lot about new scientific things, but they don't know much about the cures that Nature carries around in her saddle-bags.'

So every day the old doctor and I hunted the cure-all plant among the mountains and valleys of the Blue Ridge. Together we toiled up steep heights so slippery with fallen autumn leaves that we had to catch every sapling and branch within our reach to save us from falling. We waded through forges and chasms, breast-deep with laurel and ferns; we followed the banks of mountain streams for miles; we wound our way like Indians through brakes of pine – road-side, hill-side, river-side, mountain-side we explored in our search for the miraculous plant.

As the old doctor said, it must have grown scarce and hard to find. But we followed our quest. Day by day we plumbed the valleys, scaled the heights, and tramped the plateaux in search of the miraculous plant. Mountain bred, he never seemed to tire. I often reached home too fatigued to do anything except fall into bed and sleep until morning. This we kept up for a month.

One evening after I had returned from a six-mile tramp with the old doctor, Amaryllis and I took a little walk under the trees near the road. We looked at the mountains drawing their royal-purple robes around them for their night's repose.

'I'm glad you're well again,' she said. 'When you first came you frightened me. I thought you were really ill.'

'Well again!' I almost shrieked. 'Do you know that I have only one chance in a thousand to live?'

Amaryllis looked at me in surprise. 'Why,' said she, 'you are as strong as one of the plough-mules, you sleep ten or twelve hours every night, and you are eating us out of house and home. What more do you want?'

'I tell you,' said I, 'that unless we find the magic – that is, the plant we are looking for – in time, nothing can save me. The doctor tells me so.'

'What doctor?'

'Doctor Tatum – the old doctor who lives half-way up Black Oak Mountain. Do you know him?'

'I have known him since I was able to talk. And is that where you go every day – is it he who takes you on these long walks and climbs that have brought back your health and strength? God bless the old doctor.'

Just then the old doctor himself drove slowly down the road in his rickety old buggy. I waved my hand at him and shouted that I would be on hand the next day at the usual time. He stopped his horse and called to Amaryllis to come to him. They talked for five minutes while I waited. Then the old doctor drove on.

When we got to the house Amaryllis lugged out an encyclopædia and sought a word in it. 'The doctor said,' she told me, 'that you needn't call any more as a patient, but he'd be glad to see you any time as a friend. And then he told me to look up my name in the encyclopædia and tell you what it means. It seems to be the name of a genus of flowering plants, and also the name of a country girl in Theocritus and Virgil. What do you suppose the doctor meant by that?'

'I know what he meant,' said I. 'I know now.'

A word to a brother who may have come under the spell of the unquiet Lady Neurasthenia.

The formula was true. Even though gropingly at times, the physicians of the walled cities had put their fingers upon the specific medicament.

And so for the exercise one is referred to good Doctor Tatum on Black Oak Mountain – take the road to your right at the Methodist meeting-house in the pine-grove.

Absolute rest and exercise.

What rest more remedial than to sit with Amaryllis in the shade, and, with a sixth sense, read the wordless Theocritan idyll of the gold-bannered blue mountains marching orderly into the dormitories of the night?

Part 3: Clinical encounters

Writing prescriptions is easy, but coming to an understanding with people is hard.

Franz Kafka

From inability to let alone; from too much zeal for the new and contempt for what is old; from putting knowledge before wisdom; and science before art, and cleverness before common sense; from treating patients as cases; and from making cure of the disease more oppressive than the endurance of the same, Good Lord deliver us.

Sir Robert Hutchinson

Some patients, though concerned that their condition is perilous, recover their health simply through their contentment with the goodness of their physician.

Hippocrates (460–400 BC)

Preserve my strength, that I may be able to restore the strength of the rich and the poor, the good and the bad, the friend and the foe. Let me see in the sufferer the man alone.

Moses Maimonides (1135–1204)

Oliver Sacks

Oliver Sacks is probably the best-known physician-writer alive today. Born in London in 1933, he qualified as a doctor from Oxford University, and later emigrated to the USA where he specialised in neurology. The collections of his narratives of clinical cases – erudite, poetically written and deeply humane – have become modern classics. Of his nine books, perhaps the most famous is a collection of clinical narratives, based on his neurological cases, entitled *The Man Who Mistook His Wife For a Hat* (1985). His other books include *Awakenings* (1973), *A Leg To Stand On* (1984), *An Anthropologist on Mars* (1995), *The Island of the Color Blind* (1997) and an auto-biography, *Uncle Tungsten* (2001). Sacks still practises as a neurologist in New York, where he is a clinical professor in neurology at the Albert Einstein College of Medicine, and an adjunct professor of neurology at the NYU School of Medicine.

Oliver Sacks's stories are marked by a particular gift: the ability to see behind the masks of disease and disability, and to glimpse – with 'my human, as opposed to my neurological, vision' – the person hidden within. His stories suggest that medicine is one of the few professions where art and science can successfully combine. The story of Rebecca – the severely handicapped and disabled young woman, who yet has 'a feeling of calm and completeness, of being fully alive, of being a soul, deep and high, and equal to all others' – illustrates that fusion.

Rebecca is taken from the collection, *The Man Who Mistook His Wife For a Hat*.

Rebecca

by Oliver Sacks

Rebecca was no child when she was referred to our clinic. She was nineteen, but, as her grandmother said, 'just like a child in some ways'. She could not find her way around the block, she could not confidently open a door with a key (she could never 'see' how the key went, and never seemed to learn). She had left/right confusion, she sometimes put on her clothes the wrong way – inside out, back-to-front, without appearing to notice, or, if she noticed, without being able to get them right. She might spend hours jamming a hand or foot into the wrong glove or shoe – she seemed, as her grandmother said, to have 'no sense of space'. She was clumsy and ill-coordinated in all her movements – a 'klutz', one report said, a 'motor moron' another (although when she danced, all her clumsiness disappeared).

Rebecca had a partial cleft palate, which caused a whistling in her speech; short, stumpy fingers, with blunt, deformed nails; and a high, degenerative myopia requiring very thick spectacles – all stigmata of the same congenital condition which had caused her cerebral and mental defects. She was painfully shy and withdrawn, feeling that she was, and had always been, a 'figure of fun'.

But she was capable of warm, deep, even passionate attachments. She had a deep love for her grandmother, who had brought her up since she was three (when she was orphaned by the death of both parents). She was very fond of nature, and, if she was taken to the city parks and botanic gardens, spent many happy hours there. She was very fond too of stories, though she never learned to read (despite assiduous, and even frantic, attempts), and would implore her grandmother or others to read to her. 'She has a hunger for stories,' her grandmother said; and fortunately her grandmother loved reading stories and had a fine reading voice which kept Rebecca entranced. And not just stories – poetry too. This seemed a deep need or hunger in Rebecca – a necessary form of nourishment, of reality, for her mind. Nature was beautiful, but mute. It was not enough. She needed the world re-presented to her in verbal images, in language, and seemed to have little difficulty following the metaphors and symbols of even quite deep poems, in striking contrast to her incapacity with simple propositions and instructions. The language of feeling, of the concrete, of image and symbol formed a world she loved and, to a remarkable extent, could enter. Though conceptually (and 'propositionally') inept, she was at home with poetic language, and was herself, in a stumbling, touching way, a sort of 'primitive', natural poet. Metaphors, figures of speech, rather striking similitudes, would come naturally to her, though unpredictably, as sudden poetic ejaculations or allusions. Her grandmother was devout, in a quiet way, and this also was true of Rebecca: she loved the lighting of the Shabbath candles, the benisons and orisons which thread the Jewish day; she loved going to the synagogue, where she too was loved (and seen as a child of God, a sort of innocent, a holy fool); and she fully understood the liturgy, the chants, the prayers, rites and symbols of which the Orthodox service consists. All this was possible for her, accessible to her, loved by her, despite gross perceptual and spatio-temporal problems, and gross impairments in every schematic capacity – she could not count change, the simplest calculations defeated her, she could never learn to read or write, and she would average 60 or less in IQ tests (though doing notably better on the verbal than the performance parts of the test).

Thus she was a 'moron', a 'fool', a 'booby', or had so appeared, and so been called, throughout her whole life, but one with an unexpected, strangely moving, poetic power. Superficially she *was* a mass of handicaps and incapacities, with the intense frustrations and anxieties attendant on these; at this level she was, and felt herself to be, a mental cripple – beneath the effortless skills, the happy capacities, of others; but at some deeper level there was no sense of handicap or incapacity, but a feeling of calm and completeness, of being fully alive, of being a soul, deep and high, and equal to all others. Intellectually, then, Rebecca felt a cripple; spiritually she felt herself a full and complete being.

When I first saw her – clumsy, uncouth, all-of-a-fumble – I saw her merely, or wholly, as a casualty, a broken creature, whose neurological impairments I could pick out and dissect with precision: a multitude of apraxias and agnosias, a mass of sensorimotor impairments and breakdowns, limitations of intellectual schemata and concepts similar (by Piaget's criteria) to those of a child of eight. A poor thing, I said to myself, with perhaps a 'splinter skill', a freak gift, of speech; a mere mosaic of higher cortical functions, Piagetian schemata – most impaired.

The next time I saw her, it was all very different. I didn't have her in a test situation, 'evaluating' her in a clinic. I wandered outside, it was a lovely spring day, with a few minutes in hand before the clinic started, and there I saw Rebecca sitting on a bench, gazing at the April foliage quietly, with obvious delight. Her posture had none of the clumsiness which had so impressed me before. Sitting there, in a light dress, her face calm and slightly smiling, she suddenly brought to mind one of Chekov's young women – Irene, Anya, Sonya, Nina – seen against the backdrop of a Chekovian cherry orchard. She could have been any young woman enjoying a beautiful spring day. This was my human, as opposed to my neurological, vision.

As I approached, she heard my footsteps and turned, gave me a broad smile, and wordlessly gestured. 'Look at the world,' she seemed to say. 'How beautiful it is.' And then there came out, in Jacksonian spurts, odd, sudden, poetic ejaculations: 'spring', 'birth', 'growing', 'stirring', 'coming to life', 'seasons', 'everything in its time'. I found myself thinking of Ecclesiastes: 'To everything there is a season, and a time to every purpose under the heaven. A time to be born, and a time to die; a time to plant, and a time . . .' This was what Rebecca, in her disjointed fashion, was ejaculating – a vision of seasons, of times, like that of the Preacher. 'She is an idiot Ecclesiastes,' I said to myself. And in this phrase, my two visions of her – as idiot and as symbolist – met, collided and fused. She had done appallingly in the testing – which, in a sense, was designed, like all neurological and psychological testing, not merely to uncover, to bring out deficits, but to decompose her into functions and deficits. She had come apart, horribly, in formal testing, but now she was mysteriously 'together' and composed.

Why was she so de-composed before, how could she be so re-composed now? I had the strongest feeling of two wholly different modes of thought, or of organisation, or of being. The first schematic – pattern-seeing, problem-solving – this is what had been tested, and where she had been found so defective, so disastrously wanting. But the tests had given no inkling of anything *but* the deficits, anything, so to speak, *beyond* her deficits.

They had given me no hint of her positive powers, her ability to perceive the real world – the world of nature, and perhaps of the imagination – as a coherent, intelligible, poetic whole: her ability to see this, think this, and (when she could) live this; they had given me no intimation of her inner world, which clearly *was* composed and coherent, and approached as something other than a set of problems or tasks.

But what was the composing principle which could allow her composure (clearly it was something other than schematic)? I found myself thinking of her fondness for tales, for narrative composition and coherence. Is it possible, I wondered, that this being before me – at once a charming girl, and a moron, a cognitive mishap – can *use* a narrative (or dramatic) mode to compose and integrate a coherent world, in place of the schematic mode, which, in her, is so defective that it simply doesn't work? And as I thought, I remembered her dancing, and how this could organise her otherwise ill-knit and clumsy movements.

Our tests, our approaches, I thought, as I watched her on the bench – enjoying not just a simple but a sacred view of nature – our approach, our 'evaluations', are ridiculously inadequate. They only show us deficits, they do not show us powers; they only show us puzzles and schemata, when we need to see music, narrative, play, a being conducting itself spontaneously in its own natural way.

Rebecca, I felt, was complete and intact as 'narrative' being, in conditions which allowed her to organise herself in a narrative way; and this was something very important to know, for it allowed one to see her, and her potential, in a quite different fashion from that imposed by the schematic mode.

It was perhaps fortunate that I chanced to see Rebecca in her so-different modes – so damaged and incorrigible in the one, so full of promise and potential in the other – and that she was one of the first patients I saw in our clinic. For what I saw in her, what she showed me, I now saw in them all.

As I continued to see her, she seemed to deepen. Or perhaps she revealed, or I came to respect, her depths more and more. They were not wholly happy depths – no depths ever are – but they were predominantly happy for the greater part of the year.

Then, in November, her grandmother died, and the light, the joy, she had expressed in April now turned into the deepest grief and darkness. She was devastated, but conducted herself with great dignity. Dignity, ethical depth, was added at this time, to form a grave and lasting counterpoint to the light, lyrical self I had especially seen before.

I called on her as soon as I heard the news, and she received me, with great dignity, but frozen with grief, in her small room in the now empty house. Her speech was again ejaculated, 'Jacksonian', in brief utterances of grief and lamentation. 'Why did she have to go?' she cried; and added, 'I'm crying for me, not for her.' Then, after an interval, 'Grannie's all right. She's gone to her Long Home.' Long Home! Was this her own symbol, or an unconscious memory of, or allusion to, Ecclesiastes? 'I'm so cold,' she cried, huddling into herself. 'It's not outside, it's winter inside. Cold as death,' she added. 'She was a part of me. Part of me died with her.'

She was complete in her mourning – tragic and complete – there was absolutely no sense of her being then a 'mental defective'. After half an hour, she unfroze, regained some of her warmth and animation, said: 'It is winter. I feel dead. But I know the spring will come again.'

The work of grief was slow, but successful, as Rebecca, even when most stricken, anticipated. It was greatly helped by a sympathetic and supportive great aunt, a sister of her Grannie, who now moved into the house. It was greatly helped by the synagogue, and the religious community, above all by the rites of 'sitting shiva', and the special status accorded her as the bereaved one, the chief mourner. It was helped too perhaps by her speaking freely to me. And it was helped also, interestingly, by *dreams*, which she related with animation, and which clearly marked *stages* in the grief-work.

As I remember her, like Nina, in the April sun, so I remember her, etched with tragic clearness, in the dark November of that year, standing in a bleak cemetery in Queens, saying the Kaddish over her grandmother's grave. Prayers and Bible stories had always appealed to her, going with the happy, the lyrical, the 'blessing' side of her life. Now, in the funeral prayers, in the 103rd Psalm, and above all in the Kaddish, she found the right and only words for her comfort and lamentation.

During the intervening months (between my first seeing her, in April, and her grandmother's death that November) Rebecca – like all our 'clients' (an odious word then becoming fashionable, supposedly less degrading than 'patients'), was pressed into a variety of workshops and classes, as part of our Developmental and Cognitive Drive (these too were 'in' terms at the time).

It didn't work with Rebecca, it didn't work with most of them. It was not, I came to think, the right thing to do, because what we did was to drive them full-tilt upon their limitations, as had already been done, futilely, and often to the point of cruelty, throughout their lives.

We paid far too much attention to the defects of our patients, as Rebecca was the first to tell me, and far too little to what was intact or preserved. To use another piece of jargon, we were far too concerned with 'defectology', and far too little with 'narratology', the neglected and needed science of the concrete.

Rebecca made clear, by concrete illustrations, by her own self, the two wholly different, wholly separate, forms of thought and mind, 'paradigmatic' and 'narrative' (in Bruner's terminology). And though equally natural and native to the expanding human mind, the narrative comes first, has spiritual priority. Very young children love and demand stories, and can understand complex matters presented as stories, when their powers of comprehending general concepts, paradigms, are almost non-existent. It is this narrative or symbolic power which gives *a sense of the world* – a concrete reality in the imaginative form of symbol and story – when abstract thought can provide nothing at all. A child follows the Bible before he follows Euclid. Not because the Bible is simpler (the reverse might be said), but because it is cast in a symbolic and narrative mode.

And in this way Rebecca, at nineteen, was still, as her grandmother said, 'just like a child'. Like a child, but not a child, because she was adult. (The term 'retarded' suggests a persisting child, the term 'mentally defective' a defective adult; both terms, both concepts, combine deep truth and falsity.)

With Rebecca – and with other defectives allowed, or encouraged in, a personal development – the emotional and narrative and symbolic powers can develop strongly and exuberantly, and may produce (as in Rebecca) a sort of natural poet – or (as in José) a sort of natural artist – while the paradigmatic or conceptual powers, manifestly feeble from the start, grind very slowly and painfully along, and are only capable of a very limited and stunted development.

Rebecca realised this fully – as she had shown it to me so clearly, right from the very first day I saw her, when she spoke of her clumsiness, and of how her ill-composed and ill-organised movements became well-organised, composed and fluent, with music; and when she *showed* me how she herself was composed by a natural scene, a scene with an organic, aesthetic and dramatic unity and sense.

Rather suddenly, after her grandmother's death, she became clear and decisive. 'I want no more classes, no more workshops,' she said. 'They do nothing for me. They do nothing to bring me together.' And then, with that power for the apt model or metaphor I so admired, and which was so well developed in her despite her low IQ, she looked down at the office carpet and said:

'I'm like a sort of living carpet. I need a pattern, a design, like you have on that carpet. I come apart, I unravel, unless there's a design.' I looked down at the carpet, as Rebecca said this, and found myself thinking of Sherrington's famous image, comparing the brain/mind to an 'enchanted loom', weaving patterns ever-dissolving, but always with meaning. I thought: can one have a raw carpet without a design? Could one have the design without the carpet (but this seemed like the smile without the Cheshire cat)? A 'living' carpet, as Rebecca was, had to have both – and she especially, with her lack of schematic structure (the warp and woof, the *knit*, of the carpet, so to speak), might indeed unravel without a design (the scenic or narrative structure of the carpet).

'I must have meaning,' she went on. 'The classes, the odd jobs have no meaning . . . What I really love,' she added wistfully, 'is the theatre.'

We removed Rebecca from the workshop she hated, and managed to enroll her in a special theatre group. She loved this – it composed her; she did amazingly well: she became a complete person, poised, fluent, with style, in each role. And now if one sees Rebecca on stage, for theatre and the theatre group soon became her life, one would never even guess that she was mentally defective.

Postscript

The power of music, narrative and drama is of the greatest practical and theoretical importance. One may see this even in the case of idiots, with IQs below 20 and the extremest motor incompetence and bewilderment. Their uncouth movements may disappear in a moment with music and dancing – suddenly, with music, they know how to move. We see how the retarded, unable to perform fairly simple tasks involving perhaps four or five movements or procedures in sequence, can do these perfectly if they work to music – the sequence of movements they cannot hold as schemes being perfectly holdable as music, i.e. embedded in music. The same may be seen, very dramatically, in patients with severe frontal lobe damage and apraxia – an inability to *do* things, to retain the simplest motor sequences and programmes, even to walk, despite perfectly preserved intelligence in all other ways. This procedural defect, or motor idiocy, as one might call it, which completely defeats any ordinary system of rehabilitative instruction, vanishes at once if music is the instructor. All this, no doubt, is the rationale, or one of the rationales, of work songs.

What we see, fundamentally, is the power of music to organise – and to do this efficaciously (as well as joyfully!), when abstract or schematic forms of organisations fail. Indeed, it is especially dramatic, as one would expect, precisely when no other form of organisation will work. Thus music, or any other form of narrative, is essential when working with the retarded or apraxic – schooling or therapy for them must be centred on music or something equivalent. And in drama there is still more – there is the power of *rôle* to give organisation, to confer, while it lasts, an entire personality. The capacity to perform, to play, to *be*, seems to be a 'given' in human life, in a way which has nothing to do with intellectual differences. One sees this with infants, one sees it with the senile, and one sees it, most poignantly, with the Rebeccas of this world.

Cecil Helman

The Other Half of Eddie Barnett is based on a true case from my own clinical experience (though, of course, with names and other details changed). 'Eddie Barnett' was a puzzle to everyone, including himself, with his apparently irresolvable chronic pain: a pain both mysterious and creative. . . .

Three years after graduating from medical school in Cape Town, I had studied social anthropology at University College London, before beginning work as a family doctor in London. Anthropology – with its vivid portraits of cultural beliefs from all over the world – fascinated me, particularly its descriptions of the different types of traditional healing and exorcisms. And how so many people worldwide explained their illness by invisible entities: not called 'germs' or 'viruses', but rather malign spirits, ghosts, witches, Evil Eyes, *djinns* or *dybbuks*. At the time I was studying anthropology, I was not to know that many years later – working as a doctor in a suburban setting – some of that knowledge would come back to help me.

Even today, the case of 'Eddie Barnett' still reminds me of the comment made by the psychoanalyst Joyce McDougall, in her book *Theatres of the Body*: 'A body that suffers,' she wrote, 'is also a body that is alive.'

The Other Half of Eddie Barnett

by Cecil Helman

He had the look of a man without women. Certainly of someone who had not shared his life with a woman, for very many years.

Mr Eddie Barnett was in his late sixties, and had been divorced for about fifteen years. There were two sons living abroad, but he had virtually no contact with them.

Perhaps it was only my imagination, but he seemed to carry with him a certain dank atmosphere, a miasma of greyness and mist. His face was always long and overcast, like a late afternoon in autumn. Usually he wore a long grey coat, whatever the season, pulled over a darkish jacket which was slightly frayed at the cuffs and the collar. His mouth was turned downwards at the corners, like an inverted moon. His haircut was indifferent. His beard and moustache were ragged and streaked irregularly with grey. A deep frown divided his forehead into a grid of vertical and horizontal fissures. Under his jacket, the shirts that he wore were often crumpled, and apparently unironed. On several occasions I noticed that some of the buttons had been left undone, or had been inserted into the wrong button-hole.

Slumped over on his chair on the other side of my desk, his body collapsed into its usual heap, Mr Eddie Barnett took a deep breath. Then he gave his customary sigh, and frowned his familiar frown. The look that he fixed me with was pleading, but also accusatory.

That sigh, that misanthropic frown, those deep inhalations . . . It was not difficult to understand why so many other doctors had described him to one another as a 'heartsink' patient.

That frown, for example, always had a similar physical effect upon me. As though gravity were beckoning and all I could do was to try to stop myself sinking, thankfully, under my desk.

As usual, Eddie Barnett complained of a Pain.

But it was a pain like no other pain I had ever encountered before. It was an utterly unique pain, one that fitted no description of pain that I had ever read about, in any of my medical textbooks.

He described it always in vivid, colourful terms.

'Well, at the moment it's basically in my neck, but it often moves over to my shoulders, especially the right one. Now I can feel it in the curvature of my spine. No, no, a bit lower, more in my lower back, right near the bottom. Sometimes it moves into my stomach, here, or sometimes here, or into my bladder. But sometimes it begins to pinch on one side of my face, and then moves to the same side of my body.'

He always carried with him a full portfolio of adjectives to describe the pain. Some days it was 'sharp' and 'intense', on other days 'dull and constant' or merely a 'vague ache' or 'discomfort'. In turn it was 'heavy', 'shooting', 'burning', 'stabbing', 'shocking', or 'throbbing'. Sometimes it was accompanied by other symptoms, such as a headache (described also in equally dramatic terms), or muscular aches, or a feeling of stiffness in his neck, or shoulders, or in one leg or the other.

He was obsessed with this pain. Consultations with him always left me with a feeling of frustration, and of exhaustion. He followed every suggestion that I made with a question, and then another question after that. Asking him for more details about his pain, provoked more requests for help, and more after that. He was unsatisfiable, insatiable – like an elderly bearded baby, sucking desperately at an empty breast.

He induced in me at times (as he had in other doctors) the panicky and irrational feeling that he might never leave my room. That he might be seated there forever. That one might be trapped with him in his dolorous world, for many decades. In fact, for the rest of one's life – with nothing to look forward to except growing older, greyer, and more exhausted together – in a limbo land without hope, without any relief.

From a medical point of view, both Mr Barnett and his pain seemed to be beyond any form of palliation.

Many medical tests were carried out to discover the origin, and nature of this unusual symptom, but nothing significant was ever found. Nothing, that is, that could explain either its severity, or the complexity of its many presentations. He did of course have some physical conditions appropriate to his age, such as some osteoarthritis of his neck, but they did not match, in any proportional way, the character or intensity of the pain.

A variety of pain-killing drugs (and even, at one stage, anti-depressants) were tried, but they seemed to have no effect on the pain – or at least, only a temporary effect. In many cases, the only result of a new type of medication seemed to be for the pain to redouble its strength, almost as if it was ingesting them as a type of chemical food.

On several occasions, I offered to refer him to the counsellor, attached to our practice. She was a good listener, and skilled in understanding the inner syntax of her clients' suffering. I said that it would give him the opportunity to discuss his problems in more depth. I assured him that it would cost him nothing, and furthermore I had found out that, fortuitously, she had a vacant appointment the following week . . . As usual, he refused. What about a therapist then, at the local hospital? Also not. A psychiatrist? Oh definitely not!

'There's nothing wrong with me up here,' he said emphatically, tapping his forehead, 'I'm not mad. It's just that I've got this terrible pain that will not go away. Do you understand? It's the pain that's giving me depression. Not the other way round.'

One day, feeling particularly defeated by him, after yet another fruitless consultation, I read through the thick pile of his previous medical notes. It was a depressing, but familiar tale of medical failure. Eddie Barnett was truly a 'fat file' patient, with a thick folder filled with the frustrated letters of a dozen doctors, stretching back over many years. I noticed that the sequence of letters seemed to follow a similar pattern. First the detailed, interested letter of the keen hospital specialist, a macho young physician working in a Pain Clinic who was confident that this time he would be the one to conquer Eddie's pain. He would try one type of tablet, and then another. After the failure of several types of medications, there would be a shift to injections – sometimes of cortisone into a joint, tendon, or ligament. Then physiotherapy would be prescribed, then after that massage, acupuncture, osteopathy, and sometimes even a small machine strapped to his back which gave off an electrical signal to counter the pain. After the failure of this technique (called Transcutaneous Nerve Stimulation), a peevish tone would creep gradually into their letters. They would begin hinting at his 'emotional overlay', 'personality problems', the possibility of a 'depressive tendency'. At first this was only elliptical, but then they would blame him directly for the failure of their treatment. Eventually, they would admit defeat ('I am therefore, with some regret, referring him back to you. Perhaps you would consider referring him to a counsellor, or to a psychiatrist – ?').

As time went by, and the number of failed attempts to remove his pain accumulated, my attitude towards him underwent a gradual change. It was a slow process, and not at all conscious. My sense of irritation, and of frustration began to recede. I found myself beginning to interpret his behaviour in a rather different way. To see him, and his suffering, through a more unconventional kind of lens.

Perhaps it was because I had begun to notice something about the way he described his various, and diverse pains. Some of these, I was sure, were un-related to one another, while others did have a physical basis – but he seemed to group all of these disparate experiences into a single, painful entity. I noticed how he always described this collective essence as an 'It' – a Thing, an abstract being with its own malevolent personality. 'Now it has moved to my other shoulder', or 'Now it's going right through my chest'.

He spoke as if this 'entity' had singled him out. For reasons unknown it had chosen to enter his body and take up residence among his organs and his cells, and then torture him mercilessly for so many years. 'It is killing me', he would say, 'It is torturing me', 'It won't let me sleep at night', 'It's making me depressed', 'It's driving me mad –'.

This personalised way of talking about the pain, and its relentless attacks upon him, set me thinking. I was also struck by what seemed to be another, related pattern of behaviour. For it appeared that despite all the failed attempts at treatment, something was happening, though certainly the intensity of the pain was not improving. Something of what I had said, was being heard – at least on the bodily level. I noticed that in response to each of my suggestions – especially those that were particularly emphatic – the pain seemed for a while to go berserk. It would leap frantically around his body, like a caged animal trying to escape. It would appear first in one part of his body, then in another. Burrowing in and out of different areas of his head or chest or abdomen, with amazing rapidity – sinking then emerging, chewing its way out of this joint or that limb like a demented beaver.

I realised that Mr Barnett's syndrome need not only be interpreted using conventional medical models, or even psychological ones. As merely being an example, say, of a 'pain-prone patient' suffering from 'psychogenic pain'. On the contrary, I came to the conclusion that what he seemed to be playing out with his body, was a mystical and universal story. It was a mythology that was personal to him, and yet one that is also found in virtually every human society. It is an almost universal way of understanding suffering that would be familiar to many students of anthropology.

In trying to understand what was happening, I found myself referring, not to the medical textbooks on pain relief, but to my books on anthropology that I had studied several years before. To the voluminous literature on a particular phenomenon known as 'spirit possession'. This is the belief, found in many parts of the world, that malevolent spirits can somehow 'possess' a person – occupying their body, and causing them harm.

The anthropologist I.M. Lewis, in his book, *Ecstatic Religion*, has described dozens of cases of this belief-system from many parts of the world, but especially from Africa. He tells how in most cases an individual believes themselves to be 'possessed' against their will, by an invisible, malevolent spirit. Somehow this evil entity will 'enter' the victim's body, and then cause them to suffer illness, pain, or some other misfortune. These spirits are described as cruel and capricious, and mostly tend to strike 'without rhyme or reason'. Thus in most cases, the victim is regarded by other people as essentially innocent – since possession is often unrelated to one's prior behaviour. Sometimes, though, it is blamed on the wrath of ancestral spirits: on angry family ghosts who have been affronted by their descendant's immoral behaviour.

In some ways Eddie Barnett's pain, and the intimacy of his relationship with it, reminded me also of certain other, more specific malevolent spirits that I had read about. In the stories of Isaac Bashevis Singer, for example, the dybbuk is usually the embittered spirit of a bride or groom, who has died just before their wedding. Now it returns to 'possess' its loved one against their will, in a type of malevolent, posthumous marriage. I was also reminded of the so-called 'celestial marriage' practised in some Haitian communities (and also described by I.M. Lewis) where people about to get married go through an elaborate ceremony to first 'marry' a spirit – often that of the goddess Ezili, the patron goddess of lovers – as a way of getting protection during their real, mortal marriage.

Gradually I came to believe that the way Eddie Barnett interpreted, and described his symptoms suggested the persistence – in a diluted, Westernised form – of this ancient and pervasive mythology. That even in the present day he was, as it were, embodying this belief-system. Acting out this profound metaphor, though largely at the subconscious level.

If I was correct, and this is what was happening, then certainly Mr Eddie Barnett was a citizen of the wrong time, and the wrong place. For he was trapped in a modern, secular world where the only available exorcists were well-meaning family doctors or counsellors, or clumsy technicians in white coats who brandished stethoscopes, syringes and tablets at him – instead of feathers, drums, or holy relics.

But in his suburban milieu, on the outskirts of London, rituals of exorcism – like shamans – were in short supply. He was not religious, and belonged to no church or similar organisation. Nor was he willing to consult any of the practitioners of alternative medicine available, nor a more body-oriented psychotherapist. The only regular ritual available to him was his weekly visit to a family doctor. To a secular bespectacled healer in a secularised healing shrine. Here, in a hushed and special atmosphere, the air scented with anti-septic instead of with incense, the authentic voice of The Pain itself could at last be heard.

I began to be much more accepting of the reality of his pain – couched as it was in his chosen metaphor of malign possession. I resolved not to try, at least for a long while, to exorcise it completely from his body. For the present, his aim seemed to be to let the pain 'speak' through him, to act out its garbled message in my office in its chosen language of symptoms – and this I agreed to.

I knew also, from my studies in anthropology, that in many cases those who believe themselves to be possessed by evil spirits try to become healers them-selves. An example of this is the shaman – sometimes known as a 'master of spirits', who is able to incarnate the spirits, and then to control them. In this state of possession, the spirits are able to 'speak' through him (or her) to other people – in a spectral, distorted version of their own voice. Shamans are able to diagnose others with the same affliction, and usually to heal them by driving their spirits away. I wondered whether, in a confused and dysfunctional way, Eddie Barnett had adopted this role of oracle. It did, after all, give him a certain dignity. Perhaps he was trying to become the 'master' of his own painful spirit by giving it a voice in this way. By becoming a medium, or channeller for it, even when no-one was listening – to be a shaman without a constituency.

Quite gradually I found myself having much more respect for him, and for his predicament – though much less pity. After all, unlike many of the other people who passed through my office, Mr Barnett was never alone. However unpleasant the relationship was, he had a constant and intimate companion. His life was not as solitary as it first appeared.

Perhaps one day some patient psychoanalyst might discover the exact genealogy of the pain. Whether it was, in fact, the noxious embodiment of a punitive parent, or of an ex-wife or an absent child, or of some other demon risen from the impenetrable depths of his unconscious. I recalled that, as the psychoanalyst Joyce McDougall has put it, for some people 'physical illness may also be experienced as a reassuring proof that one's body is alive.' Perhaps that is what it was all about: for him the symptoms of pain, were also the symptoms of life. But in any case, on past experience I doubted whether he would ever accept that sort of deep psychic archaeology. In the meantime, in the rushed, and rather limited context of family medicine – all one could do was give him, and his pain, the space to be themselves. To be at least listened to sympathetically, if not placated.

It was at this point that I realised something else: something very odd about the pain itself. One day, I sat down with pen and paper, and wrote a list of all the many attributes of its complex, and rather unique 'personality' – as it had manifested itself almost weekly, in my office.

In a more traditional, primitive society prone to a belief in spirit possession, there would only be a limited number of such malign spirits available. Within each tribe, these few spirits would be fairly standardised in their behaviour. Thus their identities would be instantly recognisable by their victims, and by those around them.

However in the modern milieu in which Mr Barnett lived, with its pervasive cult of individuality, such psychological pains (or 'possessions') would tend also to be more individualistic, more personalised. In our society, their characteristics would probably be sculpted more by the individual's own psychopathology – rather than by the shared images or beliefs of their tribe.

As I wrote further, a sort of identi-kit emerged. A list of attributes of the pain, some simply descriptive, others more colourful or dramatic. Running my eye down the list before me, I soon understood why there had always been something very familiar about its particular 'personality.'

As Eddie Barnett described it – and as the pain itself spoke, indirectly, yet audibly, through him – it was actually the exact mirror-image of his own personality.

In fact, everything that Mr Eddie Barnett was, the pain was not.

And everything that he was not, the pain emphatically was.

Where Eddie Barnett was rigid, his body hardly moving beyond its tense, frozen posture – the pain was mobile. It moved here, danced there, flying swiftly from one part of the body to another, quicker than the eye could follow.

Where he was uncreative, unable to formulate new ideas or new ways of living his life – the pain was cunning and intelligent. It was endlessly creative in its invention of new forms, new appearances, new ways to dance among the cells and tendons of his body.

Where he was dull, boring, his voice flat and monotonous – the pain lived an exciting life. It clearly had a temperament that was vibrant and versatile, and full of surprises.

Where he was almost moribund, in an emotional (and social) sense – the pain was very much alive. In fact, it seemed to be looking forward to an even longer life, within its comfortable home.

Where he was frozen in his unhappiness, unable to make decisions, or decide what to do – the pain was endlessly innovative. There was no end to its ingenuity, and the strategies that it had designed to defeat the doctors.

Where he was passive, fatalistic and defeated by life and its many vicissitudes – the pain fought back. Its survival instincts were powerful, and evident, and never seemed to slacken. It was active in self-defence. It intervened in history. It outwitted – again and again – those who would have driven it out, into the wilderness.

Finally, where he was stifled and inarticulate – the pain was garrulous. Nothing could halt its talkativeness, its flow of colourful metaphors and images in its chosen language – the dialect of symptoms.

I began to stop trying to rid him of his pain. My search for new, and better, pain-killers for him became half-hearted. Instead, I began to see the world from his point of view. I sighed with him in sympathy, I frowned with him in understanding. Together we discussed the awfulness of the pain, its endless cunning, and its tenacity.

I felt that – however unsatisfactory from a medical point of view – we had developed a sort of modus vivendi. A tacit agreement. I would abandon all real attempts to destroy his pain, while he would go through the ritual of trying one pain-killer after the other, and of occasionally 'making progress' for a brief while. Our meetings took on the character of a double consultation – one with Eddie Barnett, and other with his Pain. Reassurance and explanations for Mr Barnett, some chemical food for his pain.

My exhaustion lifted, never to return. The weekly consultations with Mr Eddie Barnett and his personal dybbuk developed into a regular pattern – like a regular game of tennis, scheduled in advance. A game between two opponents who had come to know each other very well, and were equally matched. A game also that each could look forward to for the rest of the week, in anticipation of the thrill of combat – and where the score would always be one-love, or love-one, but very rarely a draw.

A sort of sad calm descended upon him. Gradually he seemed to make a melancholy peace with his invisible doppelganger, his vibrant and versatile twin. At times he seemed almost cheerful. I realised that all along I had been quite wrong about him, and his social situation: that he was not, after all, a man without a woman. On the contrary, our consultations became, increasingly, a form of marital therapy – teaching him how to live with his pain in relative harmony. And encouraging him slowly to develop – with the aid of this drug or that – a certain way of living with the dynamic, yet painful, other half of himself.

William Carlos Williams

A house call. A sick child. A battle. Doctor versus patient, child versus man. Will against will.

In writing this story, William Carlos Williams drew on his many years as a paediatrician in Rutherford, New Jersey. But he was also one of the leading American poets of his generation, as well as a novelist, essayist and playwright, and friend of many of the greatest American poets of his day, including Ezra Pound and Allen Ginsberg. In high school, Williams had already decided to become both a doctor *and* a writer, but unlike many other doctor-writers – such as Somerset Maugham, AJ Cronin and Arthur Conan Doyle – who gave up medicine for literature, Williams continued to work as a doctor for most of his life, practising in his home town until forced to stop work due to ill health.

The Use of Force recalls a deadly childhood disease, now almost forgotten. Diphtheria, often a fatal condition, was marked by fever and weakness, and by a distinctive, greyish membrane that clung to the child's tonsils.

In the encounter between the doctor and Mathilda, love and rage mingle in an intimate struggle, echoing Raphael Campo's poem, *What the Body Told*:

> I look inside their other-person's mouths
> And see the sleek interior of souls.
> It's warm and red in there – like love, with teeth.

The Use of Force

by William Carlos Williams

They were new patients to me, all I had was the name, Olson. Please come down as soon as you can, my daughter is very sick.

When I arrived I was met by the mother, a big startled looking woman, very clean and apologetic who merely said, Is this the doctor? and let me in. In the back, she added. You must excuse us, doctor, we have her in the kitchen where it is warm. It is very damp here sometimes.

The child was fully dressed and sitting on her father's lap near the kitchen table. He tried to get up, but I motioned for him not to bother, took off my overcoat and started to look things over. I could see that they were all very nervous, eyeing me up and down distrustfully. As often, in such cases, they weren't telling me more than they had to, it was up to me to tell them; that's why they were spending three dollars on me.

The child was fairly eating me up with her cold, steady eyes, and no expression to her face whatever. She did not move and seemed, inwardly, quiet; an unusually attractive little thing, and as strong as a heifer in appearance. But her face was flushed, she was breathing rapidly, and I realized that she had a high fever. She had magnificent blonde hair, in profusion. One of those picture children often reproduced in advertising leaflets and the photogravure sections of the Sunday papers.

She's had a fever for three days, began the father and we don't know what it comes from. My wife has given her things, you know, like people do, but it don't do no good. And there's been a lot of sickness around. So we tho't you'd better look her over and tell us what is the matter.

As doctors often do I took a trial shot at it as a point of departure. Has she had a sore throat?

Both parents answered me together, No . . . No, she says her throat don't hurt her.

Does your throat hurt you? added the mother to the child. But the little girl's expression didn't change nor did she move her eyes from my face.

Have you looked?

I tried to, said the mother, but I couldn't see.

As it happens we had been having a number of cases of diphtheria in the school to which this child went during that month and we were all, quite apparently, thinking of that, though no one had as yet spoken of the thing.

Well, I said, suppose we take a look at the throat first. I smiled in my best professional manner and asking for the child's first name I said, come on, Mathilda, open your mouth and let's take a look at your throat.

Nothing doing.

Aw, come on, I coaxed, just open your mouth wide and let me take a look. Look, I said opening both hands wide, I haven't anything in my hands. Just open up and let me see.

Such a nice man, put in the mother. Look how kind he is to you. Come on, do what he tells you to. He won't hurt you.

At that I ground my teeth in disgust. If only they wouldn't use the word 'hurt' I might be able to get somewhere. But I did not allow myself to be hurried or disturbed but speaking quietly and slowly I approached the child again.

As I moved my chair a little nearer suddenly with one cat-like movement both her hands clawed instinctively for my eyes and she almost reached them too. In fact she knocked my glasses flying and they fell, though unbroken, several feet away from me on the kitchen floor.

Both the mother and father almost turned themselves inside out in embarrassment and apology. You bad girl, said the mother, taking her and shaking her by one arm. Look what you've done. The nice man . . .

For heaven's sake, I broke in. Don't call me a nice man to her. I'm here to look at her throat on the chance that she might have diphtheria and possibly die of it. But that's nothing to her. Look here, I said to the child, we're going to look at your throat. You're old enough to understand what I'm saying. Will you open it now by yourself or shall we have to open it for you?

Not a move. Even her expression hadn't changed. Her breaths however were coming faster and faster. Then the battle began. I had to do it. I had to have a throat culture for her own protection. But first I told the parents that it was entirely up to them. I explained the danger but said that I would not insist on a throat examination so long as they would take the responsibility.

If you don't do what the doctor says you'll have to go to the hospital, the mother admonished her severely.

Oh yeah? I had to smile to myself. After all, I had already fallen in love with the savage brat, the parents were contemptible to me. In the ensuing struggle they grew more and more abject, crushed, exhausted while she surely rose to magnificent heights of insane fury of effort bred of her terror of me.

The father tried his best, and he was a big man but the fact that she was his daughter, his shame at her behavior and his dread of hurting her made him release her just at the critical moment several times when I had almost achieved success, till I wanted to kill him. But his dread also that she might have diphtheria made him tell me to go on, go on though he himself was almost fainting, while the mother moved back and forth behind us raising and lowering her hands in an agony of apprehension.

Put her in front of you on your lap, I ordered, and hold both her wrists.

But as soon as he did the child let out a scream. Don't, you're hurting me. Let go of my hands. Let them go I tell you. Then she shrieked terrifyingly, hysterically. Stop it! Stop it! You're killing me!

Do you think she can stand it, doctor! said the mother.

You get out, said the husband to his wife. Do you want her to die of diphtheria? Come on now, hold her, I said.

Then I grasped the child's head with my left hand and tried to get the wooden tongue depressor between her teeth. She fought, with clenched teeth, desperately! But now I also had grown furious – at a child. I tried to hold myself down but I couldn't. I know how to expose a throat for inspection. And I did my best. When finally I got the wooden spatula behind the last teeth and just the point of it into the mouth cavity, she opened up for an instant but before I could see anything she came down again and gripping the wooden blade between her molars she reduced it to splinters before I could get it out again.

Aren't you ashamed, the mother yelled at her. Aren't you ashamed to act like that in front of the doctor?

Get me a smooth-handled spoon of some sort, I told the mother. We're going through with this. The child's mouth was already bleeding. Her tongue was cut and she was screaming in wild hysterical shrieks. Perhaps I should have desisted and come back in an hour or more. No doubt it would have been better. But I have seen at least two children lying dead in bed of neglect in such cases, and feeling that I must get a diagnosis now or never I went at it again. But the worst of it was that I too had got beyond reason. I could have torn the child apart in my own fury and enjoyed it. It was a pleasure to attack her. My face was burning with it.

The damned little brat must be protected against her own idiocy, one says to one's self at such times. Others must be protected against her. It is social necessity. And all these things are true. But a blind fury, a feeling of adult shame, bred of a longing for muscular release are the operatives. One goes on to the end.

In a final unreasoning assault I overpowered the child's neck and jaws. I forced the heavy silver spoon back of her teeth and down her throat till she gagged. And there it was – both tonsils covered with membrane. She had fought valiantly to keep me from knowing her secret. She had been hiding that sore throat for three days at least and lying to her parents in order to escape just such an outcome as this.

Now truly she *was* furious. She had been on the defensive before but now she attacked. Tried to get off her father's lap and fly at me while tears of defeat blinded her eyes.

AJ Cronin

The thing's ingrained in me. It is me. I'm rotten with the rotten thing. I am the rotten thing. Rotten, I tell you.

This desperate, self-loathing cry of David Murray ('one of the best scholars that ever came out of Balliol') is the central theme of AJ Cronin's story. It is a story with strong moral undertones, a way of thinking common among doctors faced with those brought to ill health 'by their own excesses'.

AJ Cronin was born in Scotland, and qualified as a doctor from Glasgow Medical School in 1919. Later, when he began to write novels and short stories, he drew on his own medical experiences as a general practitioner in a small mining village in South Wales, and then in a fashionable practice in London's Harley Street. In 1930, he finally gave up medicine due to ill health, and from then on devoted himself entirely to writing. His most famous medical novel, *The Citadel* (1937), became a major best-seller in its day, and was later turned into a successful film. *The Citadel*'s portrayal of the inequalities in medical care is said to have helped pave the way for public acceptance of the National Health Service, ten years later.

This story is from his autobiography, *Adventures in Two Worlds* (1935), about the two worlds that he had always inhabited: medicine and literature.

The Case of David Murray

by AJ Cronin

Of all the patients who passed through my consulting-room – a long procession – none were more lamentable than those brought there by their own excesses. As I sat at my desk, my eyes shaded by my hand, listening in silence, like an *abbé* in his confessional, to some disastrous history of self-indulgence, I could not but reflect on the sweet virtue of moderation. And often, wryly, I called to memory the prophetic words of my puritanical old grandmother whose ancestor had died for the Covenant at Bothwell Bridge and who, when I was a child and detected in some misdemeanour, would call me to her knee and, having first placed her steel-rimmed spectacles in her Bible to mark the place, inform me that I should not receive from her my usual Saturday 'fairing,' then solemnly adjure me: 'You see now . . . *it pays to be good.*'

But, in this last court of appeal, when the patient was stripped for examination on my couch, it was seldom a smiling matter. There were the gluttons, the voracious eaters who, unable to resist the lure of rich meats and succulent sauces, of *pâté* and pastries and truffles, had already dug their own graves with their teeth. The old lechers, with soggy prostates, weakened sphincters, and all the load of misery which the goddess Venus joyously bestows upon her acolytes in reward for a lifetime's service. Then the drug addicts, of every shape and variety – from the pitiful old scrubwoman who used to beg tremblingly for a bottle of laudanum 'to ease her colic' – and who usually got it, poor creature – to the smart society girl, glibly sure of herself but with twitching nerves, flashing a false heroin prescription and vainly asking me to oblige her by filling it, 'as the chemist's was closed.'

Finally, there were the dipsomaniacs.

'You're wanted at once, doctor.'

'What for?'

'It's Murray, doctor. At Lee's lodging-house in the Lane.'

'I've no patient called Murray. What's the matter with him?'

'Drunk. Dead drunk again.'

'Damn it all. That's no business of mine.'

'I think it better be.' The shady-looking youth with close-cropped head and evasive eyes, who had brought the message to the surgery side door, shrugged his shoulders enigmatically. 'Or else he's sure going to croak.'

I bit my lip. How I detested these calls to Notting Hill Lane! They always meant trouble. Then, with an ill grace, I said that I would be along as soon as I was free.

Presently, then, I made my way through the nest of slums which made up the district of 'the Lane' and hammered on the blistered door of a doss-house which bore a soiled card: 'Good Beds: Men Only.' A young slattern in a shawl, who, despite the notice prohibiting her sex, seemed quite at home, admitted me.

'Murray?' I growled at her.

'All right, all right. Keep your blinking hair on. There's his room – up there.'

It was a small cubicle at the rear of the house. Because of the back-to-back construction in that congested area, the room was so dark I had to stand for a moment until my eyes adjusted themselves to the gloom. Then I made out a man lying on the torn straw mattress of a truckle bed, still wearing his clothes and boots. He was unshaven, his coat foul with mud, his collar ripped open at the neck, his eyes staring with a sort of horror into infinity. Around him was the evidence of poverty, wretchedness, misery – a bare table, an old burst trunk, a score of battered books. The squalid confusion of the room, the pitiful extremity of its occupant, forced an exclamation from me.

'My God,' I muttered involuntarily. 'What a mess!'

The sound partly roused the man upon the bed, he began to mutter incoherently to himself. He was in a thoroughly bad way, with dilated pupils, general muscular tremor, and so deeply cyanosed I could tell at once that his heart was in the Stokes-Adams syndrome. But the symptoms of delirium tremens are not particularly inspiring; I shall not dwell upon them. As I gave him a hypodermic of strychnine he raved at me feebly – the painful rhetoric of imagination driven mad by alcohol, a stream of nonsense forced from his sick, tormented mind. But as the spasm passed and he fell back exhausted on the bed, he suddenly quoted:

'*Quos deus vult perdere, prius dementat.*'

The sharp contrast from besotted ranting, the manner in which the lines were spoken took me aback. I looked at Murray more closely, trying to pierce beneath the beard and grime. He did not look old, not more than thirty-five. His hair was still thick and dark, his brow remained unlined, his features were not yet blurred or spoiled. Yet there lay upon him an air of ageless experience that was sad as death itself.

I waited until he fell into a troubled sleep, tidied up the room as best I could. I picked up a book: it was the *Aeneid*. Another: *Paolo and Francesca*. I sighed.

Then I squashed a last bug under my heel, shook myself free of fleas, listened for a moment to Murray's breathing, then stepped out of the room.

In the hallway I questioned the woman, who was waiting there. I could get nothing out of her. However, I had other sources of information and, as I was determined to learn something of my patient, I made a detour on my way home and called upon my good friend Alexander Blair.

'So you've seen Murray.' The police sergeant laid his pen on the charge desk. 'Well, there's a story there, all right. But it's a short one. Damned short. Drink.' A pause. 'Poor devil, to look at him now you wouldn't believe he'd been to Harrow and Oxford – yes, one of the best scholars that ever came out of Balliol. All sorts of things were prophesied for him – from a professorship at Oxford right up to a seat on the Woolsack. And what is he now? We've known him for about five years here, and though we had to run him in once or twice, we've done our best to give him a hand. We got him on the *Clarion* as a reporter. He did a first-class job, charmed them all for three months, then came out on his neck in the space of twenty-four hours. Faugh! It doesn't bear thinking on! Take my advice, doctor, and leave well alone.'

Nevertheless, next morning I went to see Murray again, and on several subsequent mornings. I am no altruist – visits for which I would never see my fee did not as a rule entice me. Yet something drew me to David Murray – perhaps at first his helplessness; then, later, the rare pathetic charm of the man himself.

There was no doubt of Murray's charm. Scholarly, sensitive, persuasive, witty, he was the most delightful company. As I sat listening to him I forgot the squalid room and the poverty which dwelt there – he captivated me completely.

And so it happened, one afternoon, when Murray was almost recovered from the attack and able to stagger shakily to his legs, that I braced myself and said:

'Why don't you keep off the stuff? For good, I mean. I'll do everything I can to help you.'

He stared at me sideways, then, with the first touch of bitterness he had displayed, he gave a short laugh.

'The friendship treatment, eh? You drop something in my tea when I'm not looking. Tasteless. Odourless. And I'm cured next morning. God! It's a marvellous suggestion, if only for its novelty.'

I coloured.

'I was just thinking. . . .'

'It's no good thinking, Doctor,' interposed Murray in a milder voice, 'and it's no good doing, either. Don't you think I've tried before? I've had a dozen doctors – in Liverpool, London, in Berlin, too. I've been in sanatoria till I'm sick of them. I'm the uncrowned king of inebriate homes. I've tried everything. But it's no use. The thing's ingrained in me. It is me. I'm rotten with the rotten thing. I am the rotten thing. Rotten, I tell you.' His voice rose as he went on. 'I'm a drunkard, a habitual, confirmed drunkard. The minute I'm able to leave this house I'll go round to Marney's pub. I've got my corner there. They know me. I entertain the boys. When I'm half tight I tell them bawdy stories from the French. When I'm whole tight I convulse them with Greek epigrams. They think it's Chinese – but what's the odds, they like me there. When I'm drunk, you understand. At any rate, that's where I'll go . . . and sponge on my friends. With luck I'll last six months till I get another go of d.t.'s. When the d.t.'s arrive I'm laid up for a month. My rest cure, you see. It sets me right for the next six months' drinking.'

I averted my eyes.

'If that's the way of it, then, I suppose there's nothing more to be done.'

He was silent, then a sudden impulse seemed to swing him to an opposite decision. He offered me his hand.

'Since you're so good, Doctor,' he declared, 'let's have a shot at it, for luck.'

His manner, slightly ironic, was not altogether convincing, but I could not draw back now. That same day I sent him one of my older suits, some shirts, socks, and ties, a pair of shoes and a small advance, enough to enable him to spruce himself up. Then I set about trying to find him suitable employment. It was not easy; none of the large department stores where I had hoped to place him would take him as a salesman. But finally I had a great stroke of luck.

One of my wealthier patients, Jacob Harrison, manager of the Camden Insurance Company, had a son who was preparing to take the difficult, competitive examination for entry to the Foreign Office. The boy was weak in classics and wanted someone to give him an intensive cramming for the next three months. When I mentioned that I knew of an excellent tutor, the father jumped at my suggestion. I sent David Murray along; he was interviewed and engaged.

I could not, at the outset, discern in Murray any great enthusiasm for his new position. He liked his pupil well enough and promised to pump into him an adequate amount of Euripides and Virgil, and yet there was a lack of enthusiasm, an evasiveness about him which disappointed me, made me suspect that he was not keeping his side of our pact.

But one afternoon he appeared unexpectedly at my house, burst into the consulting-room.

'Doctor,' he exclaimed, pale and breathless, 'I'm going to do it. For good this time.'

'But I thought . . . we'd agreed. . . .'

'I've been deceiving you. I haven't really been cutting it out. But now I actually mean it.'

As I gazed at him, he continued, with unmistakable determination.

'Why shouldn't I? I can do it if I want to. I've never wanted to before. But now I do. I do. Will you help me, as you said?'

'Yes,' I answered slowly, 'I'll help you.'

If there had been doubts of Murray before, now there was none – in the weeks which followed, while I stood by him, helping him as a doctor, as a friend, by every means in my power, I saw him drain the cup of suffering to the bitter dregs. In the mornings the light hurt his eyes, he felt intolerably ill, dying for a drink. He knew the agony of maddening, sleepless nights. When the craving had him by the throat he would weep from very impotence. But he held grimly on. It looked, indeed, as though he would win through at last.

Oddly enough, it had never entered my head to seek a deeper motive in Murray's struggle for redemption. But one May evening, as I stood at a window of my house, I glimpsed a situation I had not even dreamed of. Across the street, walking together, were Murray, his pupil, and a girl of nineteen whom I recognized at once as young Harrison's sister Ada, lately returned from a convent finishing school in France. There was nothing especially disturbing in the sight of these three, laughing and talking together; it was the look on Murray's face as he gazed at Ada, a look which shook me to the core.

When next I met him I mentioned, casually, the name of Ada Harrison. Immediately his face was lit by animation.

'Isn't she lovely?' he exclaimed. 'Lovelier than a rose.' And as though to himself, he murmured the line: 'Hither all dewy from her convent cell. . . .' He broke off with a smile. 'You know, Doctor, it's quite incredible. She really likes me. We walked in the park yesterday, I made her laugh at my nonsense. I could see she was enjoying herself. The first time I met her I hardly dared look at her. But now it's different. I'm beginning to find my feet again.'

It was as I had feared. He was in love. She was sweet, innocent, beautiful, and nineteen; the darling of a wealthy father. He was thirty-four, a penniless outcast, his constitution damaged beyond repair. What could one say to him? Nothing . . . nothing that would not break his heart.

Time went on. Young Harrison sat his examination and a few days later I met him in the street, in the highest spirits – he had passed well up on the list.

'We're terribly grateful to you for recommending Mr. Murray.' He beamed. 'Father wants him to take me for a vacation in France, all expenses paid. Sort of reward, you know.'

'I'm very glad for Murray's sake.'

'Oh, and by the by, Doctor, we thought, as he's almost a friend of the family now . . . we thought we'd invite him to the wedding.'

'What wedding?'

'Ada's. It's fixed for next month.' He mentioned the name of the man she was marrying, a junior partner in his father's firm, and then added, 'Your own invitation will be along quite soon.'

The invitation duly arrived. And that same evening, after my surgery, I walked slowly to Murray's lodging. I felt he might have need of my comfort and support. He was not in.

'Where can I find him?'

The woman of the house gave me her bold, scornful glance, which held now a glint of triumph.

'You might try Marney's Bar.'

Oh, no, surely not that, I thought as I hastened down the street and through the swing doors of the corner tavern. Yet it was so.

There was Murray, back in his old corner, surrounded by his coterie, swinging on his seat, blind drunk. With fumbling declamatory gestures he was quoting Homer to them: 'Gods, the old oracle returns.' And while they still sat agape, he set them guffawing with a new version of Uncle Toby and the clock. Suddenly, through the smoke, amidst the racket, his gaze caught mine. He broke off, turned clay-white, and into his eyes came the dreadful look of a soul tortured in the forsaken depths of hell.

'Curse it,' he groaned, 'why am I not dead?'

But laughter drowned the words, his glass was filled up, someone started a song. And there I had to come away and leave him.

Anton Chekhov

The setting: Lyalikov's factory outside of Moscow. Korolyov, a doctor from Moscow, arrives to visit Liza, daughter of the factory owner. She is twenty years old, sickly and frail ('The doctors say it is nerves'), but he can find nothing wrong when he examines her. In the background – in counterpoint to Liza's palpitations – the house and factory reverberate with strange, rhythmic metallic sounds. . . .

In this story, Chekhov combines acute social commentary with a deep compassion for individual suffering. Through Dr Korolyov's eyes, we glimpse some of the 'incurable illness' of industrial life: not only the inequalities, and wretchedness of the workers, but also of its effect on those who exploit them. To Korolyov, the true beneficiary of all of this is neither factory owner nor workers. 'The real person for whom everything is being done, is the devil.'

Anton Chekhov was one of the greatest Russian writers of the 19th century. He began writing stories as a medical student in Moscow, and then continued in later years while working as a doctor in remote, rural areas. He wrote many celebrated short stories, novels, essays and plays – including *Uncle Vanya*, *The Seagull* and *The Cherry Orchard*. Asked once how he could be both a doctor *and* a writer, Chekhov's famous reply was:

Medicine is my lawful wedded wife, and literature my mistress. When one gets on my nerves, I spend the night with the other. Neither one loses anything by my duplicity.

A Doctor's Visit

by Anton Chekhov

The Professor received a telegram from the Lyalikovs' factory; he was asked to come as quickly as possible. The daughter of some Madame Lyalikov, apparently the owner of the factory, was ill, and that was all that one could make out of the long, incoherent telegram. And the Professor did not go himself, but sent instead his assistant, Korolyov.

It was two stations from Moscow, and there was a drive of three miles from the station. A carriage with three horses had been sent to the station to meet Korolyov; the coachman wore a hat with a peacock's feather in it, and answered every question in a loud voice like a soldier:

'No, sir!' 'Certainly, sir!'

It was Saturday evening; the sun was setting, the work-people were coming in crowds from the factory to the station, and they bowed to the carriage in which Korolyov was driving. And he was charmed with the evening, the farmhouses and villas on the road, and the birch-trees, and the quiet atmosphere all around, when the fields and the woods and the sun seemed preparing, like the work-people now on the eve of the holiday, to rest, and perhaps to pray. . . .

He was born and had grown up in Moscow; he did not know the country, and he had never taken any interest in factories, or been inside one, but he had happened to read about factories, and had been in the houses of manufacturers and had talked to them; and whenever he saw a factory far or near, he always thought how quiet and peaceable it was outside, but within there was always sure to be impenetrable ignorance and dull egoism on the side of the owners, wearisome, unhealthy toil on the side of the work-people, squabbling, vermin, vodka. And now when the work-people timidly and respectfully made way for the carriage, in their faces, their caps, their walk, he read physical impurity, drunkenness, nervous exhaustion, bewilderment.

They drove in at the factory gates. On each side he caught glimpses of the little houses of work-people, of the faces of women, of quilts and linen on the railings. 'Look out!' shouted the coachman, not pulling up the horses. It was a wide courtyard without grass, with five immense blocks of buildings with tall chimneys a little distance one from another, warehouses and barracks, and over everything a sort of grey powder as though from dust. Here and there, like oases in the desert, there were pitiful gardens, and the green and red roofs of the houses in which the managers and clerks lived. The coachman suddenly pulled up the horses, and the carriage stopped at the house, which had been newly painted grey; here was a flower garden, with a lilac bush covered with dust, and on the yellow steps at the front door there was a strong smell of paint.

'Please come in, doctor,' said women's voices in the passage and the entry, and at the same time he heard sighs and whisperings. 'Pray walk in. . . . We've been expecting you so long . . . we're in real trouble. Here, this way.'

Madame Lyalikov – a stout elderly lady wearing a black silk dress with fashionable sleeves, but, judging from her face, a simple uneducated woman – looked at the doctor in a flutter, and could not bring herself to hold out her hand to him; she did not dare. Beside her stood a personage with short hair and a pince-nez; she was wearing a blouse of many colours, and was very thin and no longer young. The servants called her Christina Dmitryevna, and Korolyov guessed that this was the governess. Probably, as the person of most education in the house, she had been charged to meet and receive the doctor, for she began immediately, in great haste, stating the causes of the illness, giving trivial and tiresome details, but without saying who was ill or what was the matter.

The doctor and the governess were sitting talking while the lady of the house stood motionless at the door, waiting. From the conversation Korolyov learned that the patient was Madame Lyalikov's only daughter and heiress, a girl of twenty, called Liza; she had been ill for a long time, and had consulted various doctors, and the previous night she had suffered till morning from such violent palpitations of the heart, that no one in the house had slept, and they had been afraid she might die.

'She has been, one may say, ailing from a child,' said Christina Dmitryevna in a sing-song voice, continually wiping her lips with her hand. 'The doctors say it is nerves; when she was a little girl she was scrofulous, and the doctors drove it inwards, so I think it may be due to that.'

They went to see the invalid. Fully grown up, big and tall, but ugly like her mother, with the same little eyes and disproportionate breadth of the lower part of the face, lying with her hair in disorder, muffled up to the chin, she made upon Korolyov at the first minute the impression of a poor, destitute creature, sheltered and cared for here out of charity, and he could hardly believe that this was the heiress of the five huge buildings.

'I am the doctor come to see you,' said Korolyov. 'Good-evening.'

He mentioned his name and pressed her hand, a large, cold, ugly hand; she sat up, and, evidently accustomed to doctors, let herself be sounded, without showing the least concern that her shoulders and chest were uncovered.

'I have palpitations of the heart,' she said. 'It was so awful all night. . . . I almost died of fright! Do give me something.'

'I will, I will; don't worry yourself.'

Korolyov examined her and shrugged his shoulders.

'The heart is all right,' he said; 'it's all going on satisfactorily; everything is in good order. Your nerves must have been playing pranks a little, but that's so common. The attack is over by now, one must suppose; lie down and go to sleep.'

At that moment a lamp was brought into the bedroom. The patient screwed up her eyes at the light, then suddenly put her hands to her head and broke into sobs. And the impression of a destitute, ugly creature vanished, and Korolyov no longer noticed the little eyes or the heavy development of the lower part of the face. He saw a soft, suffering expression which was intelligent and touching: she seemed to him altogether graceful, feminine, and simple; and he longed to soothe her, not with drugs, not with advice, but with simple, kindly words. Her mother put her arms round her head and hugged her. What despair, what grief was in the old woman's face! She, her mother, had reared her and brought her up, spared nothing, and devoted her whole life to having her daughter taught French, dancing, music: had engaged a dozen teachers for her; had consulted the best doctors, kept a governess. And now she could not make out the reason of these tears, why there was all this misery, she could not understand, and was bewildered; and she had a guilty, agitated, despairing expression, as though she had omitted something very important, had left something undone, had neglected to call in somebody – and whom, she did not know.

'Lizanka, you are crying again . . . again,' she said, hugging her daughter to her. 'My own, my darling, my child, tell me what it is! Have pity on me! Tell me.'

Both wept bitterly. Korolyov sat down on the side of the bed and took Liza's hand.

'Come, give over; it's no use crying,' he said kindly. 'Why, there is nothing in the world that is worth those tears. Come, we won't cry; that's no good. . . .'

And inwardly he thought:

'It's high time she was married. . . .'

'Our doctor at the factory gave her kali-bromati,' said the governess, 'but I notice it only makes her worse. I should have thought that if she is given anything for the heart it ought to be drops. . . . I forget the name. . . . Convallaria, isn't it?'

And there followed all sorts of details. She interrupted the doctor, preventing his speaking, and there was a look of effort on her face, as though she supposed that, as the woman of most education in the house, she was in duty bound to keep up a conversation with the doctor, and on no other subject but medicine.

Korolyov felt bored.

'I find nothing special the matter,' he said, addressing the mother as he went out of the bedroom. 'If your daughter is being attended by the factory doctor, let him go on attending her. The treatment so far has been perfectly correct, and I see no reason for changing your doctor. Why change? It's such an ordinary trouble; there's nothing seriously wrong.'

He spoke deliberately as he put on his gloves, while Madame Lyalikov stood without moving, and looked at him with her tearful eyes.

'I have half an hour to catch the ten o'clock train,' he said. 'I hope I am not too late.'

'And can't you stay?' she asked, and tears trickled down her cheeks again. 'I am ashamed to trouble you, but if you would be so good. . . . For God's sake,' she went on in an undertone, glancing towards the door, 'do stay to-night with us! She is all I have . . . my only daughter. . . . She frightened me last night; I can't get over it. . . . Don't go away, for goodness' sake! . . .'

He wanted to tell her that he had a great deal of work in Moscow, that his family were expecting him home; it was disagreeable to him to spend the evening and the whole night in a strange house quite needlessly; but he looked at her face, heaved a sigh, and began taking off his gloves without a word.

All the lamps and candles were lighted in his honour in the drawing-room and the dining-room. He sat down at the piano and began turning over the music. Then he looked at the pictures on the walls, at the portraits. The pictures, oil-paintings in gold frames, were views of the Crimea – a stormy sea with a ship, a Catholic monk with a wine-glass; they were all dull, smooth daubs, with no trace of talent in them. There was not a single good-looking face among the portraits, nothing but broad cheekbones and astonished-looking eyes. Lyalikov, Liza's father, had a low forehead and a self-satisfied expression; his uniform sat like a sack on his bulky plebeian figure; on his breast was a medal and a Red Cross Badge. There was little sign of culture, and the luxury was senseless and haphazard, and was as uncomfortable as that uniform. The floors irritated him with their brilliant polish, the lustres on the chandelier irritated him, and he was reminded for some reason of the story of the merchant who used to go to the baths with a medal on his neck. . . .

He heard a whispering in the entry; someone was softly snoring. And suddenly from outside came harsh, abrupt, metallic sounds, such as Korolyov had never heard before, and which he did not understand now; they roused strange, unpleasant echoes in his soul.

'I believe nothing would induce me to remain here to live . . .' he thought, and went back to the music-books again.

'Doctor, please come to supper!' the governess called him in a low voice.

He went in to supper. The table was large and laid with a vast number of dishes and wines, but there were only two to supper: himself and Christina Dmitryevna. She drank Madeira, ate rapidly, and talked, looking at him through her pince-nez:

'Our work-people are very contented. We have performances at the factory every winter; the work-people act themselves. They have lectures with a magic lantern, a splendid tea-room, and everything they want. They are very much attached to us, and when they heard that Lizanka was worse they had a service sung for her. Though they have no education, they have their feelings, too.'

'It looks as though you have no man in the house at all,' said Korolyov.

'Not one. Pyotr Nikanoritch died a year and a half ago, and left us alone. And so there are the three of us. In the summer we live here, and in winter we live in Moscow, in Polianka. I have been living with them for eleven years – as one of the family.'

At supper they served sterlet, chicken rissoles, and stewed fruit; the wines were expensive French wines.

'Please don't stand on ceremony, doctor,' said Christina Dmitryevna, eating and wiping her mouth with her fist, and it was evident she found her life here exceedingly pleasant. 'Please have some more.'

After supper the doctor was shown to his room, where a bed had been made up for him, but he did not feel sleepy. The room was stuffy and it smelt of paint; he put on his coat and went out.

It was cool in the open air; there was already a glimmer of dawn, and all the five blocks of buildings, with their tall chimneys, barracks, and warehouses, were distinctly outlined against the damp air. As it was a holiday, they were not working, and the windows were dark, and in only one of the buildings was there a furnace burning; two windows were crimson, and fire mixed with smoke came from time to time from the chimney. Far away beyond the yard the frogs were croaking and the nightingales singing.

Looking at the factory buildings and the barracks, where the work-people were asleep, he thought again what he always thought when he saw a factory. They may have performances for the work-people, magic lanterns, factory doctors, and improvements of all sorts, but, all the same, the work-people he had met that day on his way from the station did not look in any way different from those he had known long ago in his childhood, before there were factory performances and improvements. As a doctor accustomed to judging correctly of chronic complaints, the radical cause of which was incomprehensible and incurable, he looked upon factories as something baffling, the cause of which also was obscure and not removable, and all the improvements in the life of the factory hands he looked upon not as superfluous, but as comparable with the treatment of incurable illnesses.

'There is something baffling in it, of course . . .' he thought, looking at the crimson windows. 'Fifteen hundred or two thousand work-people are working without rest in unhealthy surroundings, making bad cotton goods, living on the verge of starvation, and only waking from this nightmare at rare intervals in the tavern; a hundred people act as overseers, and the whole life of that hundred is spent in imposing fines, in abuse, in injustice, and only two or three so-called owners enjoy the profits, though they don't work at all, and despise the wretched cotton. But what are the profits, and how do they enjoy them? Madame Lyalikov and her daughter are unhappy – it makes one wretched to look at them; the only one who enjoys her life is Christina Dmitryevna, a stupid, middle-aged maiden lady in pince-nez. And so it appears that all these five blocks of buildings are at work, and inferior cotton is sold in the Eastern markets, simply that Christina Dmitryevna may eat sterlet and drink Madeira.'

Suddenly there came a strange noise, the same sound Korolyov had heard before supper. Someone was striking on a sheet of metal near one of the buildings; he struck a note, and then at once checked the vibrations, so that short, abrupt, discordant sounds were produced, rather like 'Dair . . . dair . . . dair. . . .' Then there was half a minute of stillness, and from another building there came sounds equally abrupt and unpleasant, lower bass notes: 'Drin . . . drin . . . drin. . . .' Eleven times. Evidently it was the watchman striking the hour.

Near the third building he heard: 'Zhuk . . . zhuk . . . zhuk. . . .' And so near all the buildings, and then behind the barracks and beyond the gates. And in the stillness of the night it seemed as though these sounds were uttered by a monster with crimson eyes – the devil himself, who controlled the owners and the work-people alike, and was deceiving both.

Korolyov went out of the yard into the open country.

'Who goes there?' someone called to him at the gates in an abrupt voice.

'It's just like being in prison,' he thought, and made no answer.

Here the nightingales and the frogs could be heard more distinctly, and one could feel it was a night in May. From the station came the noise of a train; somewhere in the distance drowsy cocks were crowing; but, all the same, the night was still, the world was sleeping tranquilly. In a field not far from the factory there could be seen the framework of a house and heaps of building material: Korolyov sat down on the planks and went on thinking.

'The only person who feels happy here is the governess, and the factory hands are working for her gratification. But that's only apparent: she is only the figurehead. The real person, for whom everything is being done, is the devil.'

And he thought about the devil, in whom he did not believe, and he looked round at the two windows where the fires were gleaming. It seemed to him that out of those crimson eyes the devil himself was looking at him – that unknown force that had created the mutual relation of the strong and the weak, that coarse blunder which one could never correct. The strong must hinder the weak from living – such was the law of Nature; but only in a newspaper article or in a school book was that intelligible and easily accepted. In the hotchpotch which was everyday life, in the tangle of trivialities out of which human relations were woven, it was no longer a law, but a logical absurdity, when the strong and the weak were both equally victims of their mutual relations, unwillingly submitting to some directing force, unknown, standing outside life, apart from man.

So thought Korolyov, sitting on the planks, and little by little he was possessed by a feeling that this unknown and mysterious force was really close by and looking at him. Meanwhile the east was growing paler, time passed rapidly; when there was not a soul anywhere near, as though everything were dead, the five buildings and their chimneys against the grey background of the dawn had a peculiar look – not the same as by day; one forgot altogether that inside there were steam motors, electricity, telephones, and kept thinking of lake-dwellings, of the Stone Age, feeling the presence of a crude, unconscious force. . . .

And again there came the sound: 'Dair . . . dair . . . dair . . . dair . . .' twelve times. Then there was stillness, stillness for half a minute, and at the other end of the yard there rang out:

'Drin . . . drin . . . drin. . . .'

'Horribly disagreeable,' thought Korolyov.

'Zhuk . . . zhuk . . .' there resounded from a third place, abruptly, sharply, as though with annoyance – 'Zhuk . . . zhuk. . . .'

And it took four minutes to strike twelve. Then there was a hush; and again it seemed as though everything were dead.

Korolyov sat a little longer, then went to the house, but sat up for a good while longer. In the adjoining rooms there was whispering, there was a sound of shuffling slippers and bare feet.

'Is she having another attack?' thought Korolyov.

He went out to have a look at the patient. By now it was quite light in the rooms, and a faint glimmer of sunlight, piercing through the morning mist, quivered on the floor and on the wall of the drawing-room. The door of Liza's room was open, and she was sitting in a low chair beside her bed, with her hair down, wearing a dressing-gown and wrapped in a shawl. The blinds were down on the windows.

'How do you feel?' asked Korolyov.

'Thank you.'

He touched her pulse, then straightened her hair, that had fallen over her forehead.

'You are not asleep,' he said. 'It's beautiful weather outside. It's spring. The nightingales are singing, and you sit in the dark and think of something.'

She listened and looked into his face; her eyes were sorrowful and intelligent, and it was evident she wanted to say something to him.

'Does this happen to you often?' he said.

She moved her lips, and answered:

'Often, I feel wretched almost every night.'

At that moment the watchman in the yard began striking two o'clock. They heard: 'Dair . . . dair . . .' and she shuddered.

'Do those knockings worry you?' he asked.

'I don't know. Everything here worries me,' she answered, and pondered. 'Everything worries me. I hear sympathy in your voice; it seemed to me as soon as I saw you that I could tell you all about it.'

'Tell me, I beg you.'

'I want to tell you my opinion. It seems to me that I have no illness, but that I am weary and frightened, because it is bound to be so and cannot be otherwise. Even the healthiest person can't help being uneasy if, for instance, a robber is moving about under his window. I am constantly being doctored,' she went on, looking at her knees, and she gave a shy smile. 'I am very grateful, of course, and I do not deny that the treatment is a benefit; but I should like to talk, not with a doctor, but with some intimate friend who would understand me and would convince me that I was right or wrong.'

'Have you no friends?' asked Korolyov.

'I am lonely. I have a mother; I love her, but, all the same, I am lonely. That's how it happens to be. . . . Lonely people read a great deal, but say little and hear little. Life for them is mysterious; they are mystics and often see the devil where he is not. Lermontov's Tamara was lonely and she saw the devil.'

'Do you read a great deal?'

'Yes. You see, my whole time is free from morning till night. I read by day, and by night my head is empty; instead of thoughts there are shadows in it.'

'Do you see anything at night?' asked Korolyov.

'No, but I feel. . . .'

She smiled again, raised her eyes to the doctor, and looked at him so sorrowfully, so intelligently; and it seemed to him that she trusted him, and that she wanted to speak frankly to him, and that she thought the same as he did. But she was silent, perhaps waiting for him to speak.

And he knew what to say to her. It was clear to him that she needed as quickly as possible to give up the five buildings and the million if she had it – to leave that devil that looked out at night; it was clear to him, too, that she thought so herself, and was only waiting for someone she trusted to confirm her.

But he did not know how to say it. How? One is shy of asking men under sentence what they have been sentenced for; and in the same way it is awkward to ask very rich people what they want so much money for, why they make such a poor use of their wealth, why they don't give it up, even when they see in it their unhappiness; and if they begin a conversation about it themselves, it is usually embarrassing, awkward, and long.

'How is one to say it?' Korolyov wondered. 'And is it necessary to speak?'

And he said what he meant in a roundabout way:

'You in the position of a factory owner and a wealthy heiress are dissatisfied; you don't believe in your right to it; and here now you can't sleep. That, of course, is better than if you were satisfied, slept soundly, and thought everything was satisfactory. Your sleeplessness does you credit; in any case, it is a good sign. In reality, such a conversation as this between us now would have been unthinkable for our parents. At night they did not talk, but slept sound; we, our generation, sleep badly, are restless, but talk a great deal, and are always trying to settle whether we are right or not. For our children or grandchildren that question – whether they are right or not – will have been settled. Things will be clearer for them than for us. Life will be good in fifty years' time; it's only a pity we shall not last out till then. It would be interesting to have a peep at it.'

'What will our children and grandchildren do?' asked Liza.

'I don't know. . . . I suppose they will throw it all up and go away.'

'Go where?'

'Where? . . . Why, where they like,' said Korolyov; and he laughed. 'There are lots of places a good, intelligent person can go to.'

He glanced at his watch.

'The sun has risen, though,' he said. 'It is time you were asleep. Undress and sleep soundly. Very glad to have made your acquaintance,' he went on, pressing her hand. 'You are a good, interesting woman. Good-night!'

He went to his room and went to bed.

In the morning when the carriage was brought round they all came out on to the steps to see him off. Liza, pale and exhausted, was in a white dress as though for a holiday, with a flower in her hair; she looked at him, as yesterday, sorrowfully and intelligently, smiled and talked, and all with an expression as though she wanted to tell him something special, important – him alone. They could hear the larks trilling and the church bells pealing. The windows in the factory buildings were sparkling gaily, and, driving across the yard and afterwards along the road to the station, Korolyov thought neither of the workpeople nor of lake dwellings, nor of the devil, but thought of the time, perhaps close at hand, when life would be as bright and joyous as that still Sunday morning; and he thought how pleasant it was on such a morning in the spring to drive with three horses in a good carriage, and to bask in the sunshine.

Moacyr Scliar

Moacyr Scliar is one of the best-known writers in Brazil. He is also a public health physician. His many books – novels, short stories, essays, non-fiction – are written with great imaginative power, and several of them blend Brazilian and Jewish themes. Among his best-known works are the collection of short stories *O Carnaval dos Animais* (*The Carnival of the Animals*) and the novel *O Centauro no Jardin* (*The Centaur in the Garden*) – both written in a style often called 'magical realism'.

This extract comes from his *A Majestade do Xingu* (*The King of Xingu*), published in 1997. The book has been highly praised, receiving the Brazilian Academy of Letters's prize for the best Brazilian novel of 1997. It is a fictionalised account of the life of Noel Nutels, a Jewish doctor born in 1913 in Ananiev, Ukraine, and who came as a boy to Brazil. After qualifying in medicine in Recife in 1938, he dedicated his life to taking care of the indigenous Indians in the region of Xingu, in the remote hinterland of Brazil.

The following extract describes the first contact between Nutels and the local Kalapalo Indians. It tells of the clash of two perspectives: that of modern, scientific medicine and the older, traditional remedies of the local *xaman*, or indigenous healer. For the Kalapalo, the defeat of their *xaman* marks the arrival of a new form of healing: efficient, but impersonal; rooted in science, rather than in nature.

The King of Xingu

by Moacyr Scliar

The Kalapalo look at him with great curiosity and puzzlement.

The interpreter says Noel is a physician sent by the government to protect Indians from many diseases, to cure them. The Kalapalo listen with great attention. The interpreter talks for a long time. Afterwards silence. Only the wind in the trees, a bird singing in the forest.

The chief of the Indians, the *cacique*, a short but strong man says something in a guttural voice. The interpreter listens carefully. Then he translates to Noel: there is a sick girl in the village, the Indians did everything they could but she got worse; they ask if you can treat her. And after a pause he adds:

– 'I think they want to see if white medicine really works. It is a test for you'.

Noel is a doctor. Not much of a doctor, according to some of his colleagues; he is a Public Health physician which means, for them, that he is not able to treat sick people. He can treat the social body, but at this moment it is not the social body which is diseased, it's the body of a small girl. Is he prepared for it? He's not sure, but he cannot hesitate:

– 'Let's go'.

The Indians take him to a small hut made of branches. There, lying on a mat is the girl. She's about ten and it's not necessary to be a doctor to realise she's very ill. Sweat covers her body, she breathes quickly and with difficulty, her abdomen is distended. A woman, the girl's mother, says something that the interpreter translates: she's been ill for several days but got much worse in the last hours.

Noel kneels and looks at the girl. Yes, he saw this situation a couple of times before: sweating, shallow breathing, a protruding abdomen ... It's not an unknown situation.

Never mind, he has to do something. This is what the Indians expect from him: that he will do something. He decides to use penicillin. He opens his bag, finds the flask with the white powder, the vial with distilled water and the syringe. He prepares the solution and injects it in the arm of the girl. Who suddenly awakens from the torporous state, grabs the hand of Noel and bites it furiously. The Indians laugh: not only do they love to see a white man scared but they also feel relieved: if the girl is biting, it's because she's probably better.

With a gauze, Noel cleans the blood off his hand. He also feels relieved. Biting is a form of acceptance. Between her teeth the girl has, by now, small fragments of his tissues. The particles of those tissues will soon be part of her body. A small, gentle anthropophagy, which, in a way, redeems him.

Now we have to wait, he says, and the interpreter translates. The *cacique* invites both men to eat. The food is served in a kind of basket, some dark powder. Roasted, ground up grasshoppers. It is very difficult to eat, but Noel cannot refuse. Then he offers cream crackers to the Indians. They taste it and spit: obviously they don't like that white man's food.

Noel spends all night and the following day in the hut with the little girl and her mother. He injects penicillin, he checks her temperature, he looks in her face for signs of improvement. This is what finally happens: the girl has no fever anymore, she's smiling and asking for food.

Six o'clock in the afternoon. Noel gets out of the hut and walks to the river and looks at the majestic Xingu flowing through the forest. It was a long way, from Ananiev, the Jewish village in Russia to this place. But now he, Noel Nutels, is part of this scenario, like the Indians. Now he is entirely Brazilian. And he is happy.

But someone is not happy. The *xaman*, the medicine man of the Kalapalo. An old man, he was the one the Indians looked for in case of disease. Now there is this white doctor, with his strong medicines. The *xaman* observed from the hut's door what Noel did. It's something mysterious for him, but undoubtedly it's strong medicine, the white powder, much stronger than his herbs or songs. And it's stronger mainly because it's white. The *xaman* is afraid of white. White denies all colours, the green of the forest, the blue of the sky, the yellow of the flowers. White is white, and white is powerful. From now on, for any disease, the Indians will prefer the white powder. He, the *xaman*, will be no longer necessary. Unless –

Unless he kills the enemy. By sorcery, of course he's not a murderer. But he knows some powerful forms of sorcery; which he learned from his father, also a *xaman*. And No, he won't do it. First of all, he is not sure that sorcery will work against this powerful white man. If he can cure diseases, he can also, and easily, protect himself against sorcery. It will be another defeat for the *xaman*.

No he must go. He must realise that his time is over. The time for herbs, for magic songs, for sorcery, is over. Now it's the time for white powder. Now it is the time for white doctors, for white men. He must depart, and he will depart. Hoping, deep in his heart, that some day the white medicine, the white powder, will fail. The Kalapalo will look for him and he will return, in glory, to treat the diseased Indian bodies with herbs and magic songs.

Notes on the contributors

Mikhail Bulgakov was born in 1891 in Kiev, Ukraine, and graduated as a doctor there in 1916. As an alternative to military service, he worked in remote rural hospitals for two years – which provided the material for *A Country Doctor's Notebook* – and then for a while as a venereologist in Kiev. His first book, serialised in 1924, was *Belaya gvardiya* (*The White Guard*). He wrote plays, novels and a biography of Molière. Accused by the authorities in the 1930s of 'slandering Soviet reality', he was prevented from having his books published. His most famous novel, *The Master and Margarita*, was published posthumously. He died in Moscow in 1940.

Anton Chekhov, born in 1860, was one of the most celebrated Russian writers of the 19th century. In 1884 he graduated from the Medical Faculty of Moscow University, and for most of his life practised as a doctor, mainly in rural areas. During the terrible 1891–92 famine he worked on disaster relief. He wrote novels, essays, short stories and plays, including *Uncle Vanya*, *The Seagull* and *The Cherry Orchard*. Chekhov died of tuberculosis in 1904.

Rachel Clark was born in 1970 in London, England. She was educated at the University of Bristol, where she studied psychology, and then trained as an occupational therapist, before working as a management consultant. At the age of 25, while working for two years in Australia, she was diagnosed as having a rare head and neck cancer. She was treated initially in Sydney, then back in London. After her return to the UK in 1996, she began to write a detailed account of her experiences of the disease. She died in 1998. Her book *A Long Walk Home* (2002) includes an Epilogue by her twin sister, Naomi Jefferies.

AJ Cronin was born in Scotland in 1896, and qualified as a doctor from Glasgow Medical School in 1919. He worked as a ship's doctor, then as a general practitioner in South Wales, later moving to London. In 1930, he gave up medicine due to ill health, and from then on devoted himself to writing. Among his most famous books are *The Citadel* (1937) and *The Keys of the Kingdom* (1942), and the autobiographical *Adventures in Two Worlds* (1935). He died in 1981.

Arthur Conan Doyle was born in Scotland in 1859, and qualified as a doctor at the University of Edinburgh in 1881. At various times he worked as a ship's doctor, a general physician, an eye specialist and the director of a military hospital. In 1890, he gave up medicine to write full time, and is most famous for his Sherlock Holmes stories and his historical novels. His book of short stories, *Tales of Adventure and Medical Life*, was first published in 1922. He died in 1930.

Cecil Helman was born in 1944 in Cape Town, South Africa, where he qualified as a doctor. In 1969 he moved to London, where he studied social anthropology at University College London. He has written short stories, prose poems, essays and travel pieces. His books include *Body Myths* (published in the USA as *The Body of Frankenstein's Monster: essays in myth and medicine*), *The Exploding Newspaper & Other Fables* and a textbook, *Culture, Health and Illness*. His work has been translated into six languages. He lives in London.

O Henry was the pseudonym of William Sydney Porter, born in 1862 in Greenboro, North Carolina, the son of a physician. During his life, he published ten collections of short stories, a total of 300 stories in all. These collections include *Cabbages and Kings* (1904), *The Four Million* (1906) and *The Trimmed Lamp* (1907). His most famous story is probably *The Gift of the Magi*. O Henry's life was overshadowed by alcoholism, ill health and financial problems – and by three years spent in jail for embezzlement. He died in 1910.

Franz Kafka was born in Prague in 1883. He began studying literature and medicine for a short time, but then turned to law, obtaining his doctorate from Prague University. Later he worked for many years in an insurance company. Although a Czech, his novels, short stories and parables were all written in German. He died of tuberculosis in 1924. Some of his most famous books were published posthumously, including *The Trial* (1925), *The Castle* (1926), *America* (1927) and *The Great Wall of China* (1931).

W Somerset Maugham was born in Paris in 1874. He qualified as a doctor at St Thomas' Hospital, London, in 1897, and practised for a while in London's East End, before giving up medicine for writing. His first novel, *Liza of Lambeth* (1897), was based on these early medical experiences, while his most famous novel, *Of Human Bondage*, also had a medical protagonist – Philip Carey, born with a clubfoot, who studies art and then becomes a doctor. He wrote novels, plays, short stories and travel pieces. He died in 1965.

Ruth Picardie was born in 1964 in Reading, England. She studied social anthropology at Cambridge University, and then worked as a journalist and freelance writer. In 1996, she was diagnosed as having breast cancer, from which she died in 1998. In her last year, she wrote five columns on her illness in the *Life* magazine of the *Observer* newspaper, and also had an extensive e-mail correspondence with friends and well-wishers. After her death, these columns and e-mails were collected into a book – *Before I Say Goodbye* (1998) – by her husband and sister.

Rachel Naomi Remen, a cancer specialist and therapist, is a pioneer of the holistic and more spiritual approach to healthcare – especially in life-threatening diseases. Her books include *Kitchen Table Wisdom: stories that heal* and *My Grandfather's Blessings: stories of strength, refuge and belonging.* She is a clinical professor of family and community medicine at the University of California, San Francisco.

Renate Rubinstein was born in 1929 in Berlin, but moved to Holland with her family in 1935. During the Second World War, her father was killed at Auschwitz. For many years she worked as a columnist on the Amsterdam weekly newspaper *Vrij Nederland*, writing under the pseudonym 'Tamar', and was the author of 20 books on various social and political topics. At the age of 47 she was diagnosed as suffering from multiple sclerosis, and her book *Take It and Leave It* is a record of her experiences. She died in Amsterdam in 1990.

Oliver Sacks was born in London in 1933. He obtained his medical degree from Oxford University in 1958, and later emigrated to the USA where he specialised in neurology. He has published nine books, which have been translated into 22 languages. The collections of his clinical narratives – poetically written, and deeply humane – have become modern classics, and include *Awakenings* (1973), *A Leg To Stand On* (1984), *The Man Who Mistook His Wife For a Hat* (1985), *An Anthropologist on Mars* (1995) and *The Island of the Color Blind* (1997). He has also published an autobiography, *Uncle Tungsten* (2001). He lives in New York.

Moacyr Scliar was born in 1937 in Porto Alegre, in the state of Rio Grande do Sul, Brazil, where he qualified as a doctor in 1962. He has worked for many years as a public health doctor. He is one of Brazil's leading writers, author of many imaginative novels and short stories, and recipient of many literary prizes. Among his best-known novels are: *O Carnaval dos Animais* (*The Carnival of the Animals*) and *O Centauro no Jardin* (*The Centaur in the Garden*). His novel *A Majestade do Xingu* (*The King of Xingu*), received the Brazilian Academy of Letters's prize for the best Brazilian novel of 1997. He lives in Porto Alegre.

Clive Sinclair was born in 1948 in London, and educated at the University of East Anglia and the University of California at Santa Cruz. He is the author of five novels and three collections of stories, including *Blood Libels* (1985), *The Lady with the Laptop* (1996), which won PEN Silver Pen Award, *A Soap Opera*

From Hell (1998) and *Meet the Wife* (2002). His first book of stories, *Hearts of Gold*, won the Somerset Maugham Award. From 1983 to 1987 he was the literary editor of the London *Jewish Chronicle*. He lives in St Albans, England.

William Carlos Williams was born in 1883, and graduated as a doctor from the University of Pennsylvania in 1906. For most of his working life he worked as a paediatrician in his home town of Rutherford, New Jersey. He became one of the leading American poets, and also wrote novels, plays, short stories and essays. During his life he received many awards, and was a friend of many famous American poets, including Ezra Pound and Allen Ginsberg. He died in 1963.

Note: I am indebted for some of this information to the *Roster of Physician Writers* website (http://members.aol.com/dbryantmd), compiled by Daniel C Bryant MD, which includes brief biographical – and bibliographical – details of over 300 physician-writers.

Further reading

Bell C (1984) A hundred years of Lancet language. *Lancet*. **ii**: 1453.

Belli A and Coulehan J (eds) (1998) *Blood and Bone: poems by physicians*. University of Iowa Press.

Brody H (1987) *Stories of Sickness*. Yale University Press.

Bulgakov M (1975) *A Country Doctor's Notebook*. Collins & Harvill.

Cassell EJ (1976) *The Healer's Art*. JB Lippincott.

Clark R (2002) *A Long Walk Home*. Radcliffe Medical Press.

Coles R (1984) *The Doctor Stories*. New Directions.

Coope R (1952) *The Quiet Art: a doctor's anthology*. E & S Livingstone.

Cousins N (1979) *Anatomy of an Illness as Perceived by the Patient*. WW Norton.

Cousins N (1982) *The Physician and Literature*. Saunders.

Crichton M (1988) *Travels*. Pan Books.

Crichton M (1995) *Five Patients*. Arrow.

Cronin AJ (1937) *The Citadel*. Gollancz.

Cronin AJ (1952) *Adventures in Two Worlds*. Gollancz.

Doyle AC (1963) *Tales of Adventure and Medical Life*. John Murray.

Gordon R (1993) *The Literary Companion to Medicine: an anthology of prose and poetry*. Sinclair-Stevenson.

Grouse LD (1983) Has the machine become the physician? *Journal of the American Medical Association*. **250**: 1891.

Helman C (1992) *The Body of Frankenstein's Monster: essays in myth and medicine*. WW Norton.

Helman C (2001) *Culture, Health and Illness* (4e). Arnold.

Henry O (1954) *The Best of O Henry: chosen by Sapper*. Hodder and Stoughton.

Kaufman SR (1993) *The Healer's Tale*. University of Wisconsin Press.

Kleinman A (1988) *The Illness Narratives*. Basic Books.

Konner M (1993) *The Trouble With Medicine*. BBC Books.

Mann T (1969) *The Magic Mountain*. Random House.

McDougall J (1989) *Theatres of the Body*. Free Association Books.

Muir Gray JA (1999) Postmodern medicine. *Lancet*. **354**: 1550–3.

Picardie R (with Matt Seaton and Justine Picardie) (1998) *Before I Say Goodbye*. Penguin Books.

Porter R (ed.) (1985) *Patients and Practitioners*. Cambridge University Press.

Remen RN (1996) *Kitchen Table Wisdom*. Riverhead Books.

Remen RN (2000) *My Grandfather's Blessings*. Riverhead Books.

Rubinstein R (1985) *Take It and Leave It*. Marion Boyars.

Sacks O (1985) *The Man Who Mistook His Wife For a Hat*. Picador.

Sacks O (1991) *A Leg To Stand On* (revised edition). Picador.

Selzer R (1982) *Confessions of a Knife*. Triad/Granada.

Sinclair C (1998) *A Soap Opera From Hell*. Picador.

Sontag S (1978) *Illness as Metaphor*. Vintage.

Tudor Hart J (1988) *A New Kind of Doctor*. Merlin Press.